EXECUTE

EXECUTE

A guide for your journey towards the most powerful version of you. Take courage to love.

Copyright © 2019 Regina Stump

All rights reserved.

ISBN: *9781712166185*

Imprint: *Independently published*

To the only other Leader I would follow into battle; Believe in you as much as I do.

Regina Stump

TABLE OF CONTENTS

Prologue	*vi*
Chapter 1	*1*
Chapter 2	*14*
Chapter 3	*22*
Chapter 4	*29*
Chapter 5	*38*
Chapter 6	*46*
Chapter 7	*56*
Chapter 8	*78*
Chapter 9	*91*
Chapter 10	*102*
Chapter 11	*114*
Chapter 12	*126*
Chapter 13	*136*
Chapter 14	*145*
Chapter 15	*162*
Epilogue	*169*
About the Author	*175*

"To win, you have to execute. Execution requires readiness. Readiness is no accident" (Zigarelli, 2011, p. 83).

"To live a life of purpose, influence , and leadership, one must love. One must choose to love the power of choice, the power of free will, the power of relationship. Purpose is a product of the execution of excellence driven by love. Preparation of purpose requires practice of execution" (Me, 2019).

To my heroes of inspiration:

Tracy. Thank you for being pure and beautiful life, for being joy, and for being the catalyst for this work. I love you more than words. You'll always be older than me.

Dad. Thank you for being my hero, and for your unceasing support of my endeavors. This specific one didn't include dirt or sandbag marches. Thank you for loving me unconditionally, and for being an unwavering example of servant leadership and hard work.

Sage, Tori, & Mom. Thank you for being my spark, my cheering section when I doubted myself. Thank you for never taking it easy on me. Thank you for loving me always, despite my constant shenanigans. Thank you for loving me graciously through my struggles, and during the moments when I was tough to love. Thank you for fighting for me.

Janice and Larry. Thank you for carting "The Kid's" sorry butt around when I was unable to drive. You are an answer to prayer; and you are more meaningful than you'll ever know. See you at the crack of dawn, walking with Sadie.

Diana and Jonny; and Peanut. Thank you for allowing me to be your personal trainer, for putting up with my quirks, and for making you do burpees. Thank you for encouraging me, for supporting me, and for sharing your wisdom and experiences. Thank you for caring about me. Thank you for your love for each other, and for life. And thank you for having the best doggo.

Janet and Rich. Thank you for your generosity; your care, and your knowledge. Thank you for rearranging your life on my behalf.

Thank you doesn't go nearly far enough. I hope to one day express my gratitude in ways over simple words.

Friends, Neighbors, Mentors. Thank you for your investment into my life. Your presence and your thoughts, no matter how seemingly insignificant, mean more than you'll realize. You each have played a vital role in my life. Thank you for going above and beyond, in order to care for me. I am blessed, and I am grateful for you.

Coach. Thank you for the program at Messiah you have developed; centered on Christ. Thank you for preparing and equipping athletes to step into the real world with qualities gained trough sport. Thank you for your role in my life and in my character development. Thank you for your for mentorship. I would not be here without you. I would not be here without those many miles run. Or those Peanut M&Ms.

PROLOGUE

The words of this novel are for you to interpret, to laugh at, to mull over, or even to use as toilet paper if you so choose. The personal stories I share and the themes that I highlight are intended to be useful. By no means do my acclamations matter for this novel. My athletic and academic achievements are to serve as proof, as personal demonstration, for your understanding of context and application. My words mean nothing without evidence. Proof of my habits and pursuit of health diminish in meaning should I need to elucidate them with words.

Other than my fondness for unicorns, I am nothing extraordinary. I seek health and success just like you. I struggle with relationships. I work hard, but I still fail. I am human.

I am an athlete; I am competitive. I seek to abolish "good enough". I put 100% of my entire being into all endeavors I pursue. I find energy in the risk of failure. I search for discomfort. I push boundaries. Who I am is reflected in how I express myself. The words and experiences that I share are meant for you. My common life, yet unique experiences, have given me perspective that can be adopted by you. What I have done, experiences I have been through, and adventures around the world mean little. My meaning and my "why" that drives who I am, is a source of life and love. Life, power, excellence, and love are why we exist. You possess them. You matter. Your meaning can only be fulfilled by you.

The words you read are to inspire; to initiate a stirring in your soul. Go. Be. Execute a course of action.

Words without action are meaningless.

My hope is that you choose embrace these words, and thus, execute.

Execute… how?

Read on.

And take charge of your path ahead, with the dominance of a lion.

Take courage.

You may need it, should you venture to convert these words into action.

Be courageous, and with the boldness of a lion, turn the page.

CHAPTER 1

CHAMPION. CHALLENGE. CHOICE.

One in heart and mind. Two National Championships. Four years of the toughest and most rewarding experiences as an NCAA women's soccer athlete. One small college in the middle of cornfields and mountains of Pennsylvania. A host of relationships that impacted me more than words can describe. I am who I am today because of Messiah Women's Soccer.

The expectations of playing soccer were founded on the pursuit of excellence. In every pursuit- athletically, personally, academically- excellence was the driving force. The standard was characterized as behavior above reproach. Messiah Women's Soccer (MWS) was built on the framework of several key elements and principles:

- The team comes first. There is no place for selfishness, egotism, or envy
- We have complete control over our physical preparation and take responsibility for it
- We choose to be positive

- There are no unimportant details. We do things a certain way for a reason. "Little things make big things happen"
- We mean no offense and take no offense with each other
- Team Spirit: Eagerness to sacrifice personal interests of glory for the welfare of all
- Success: Giving of your best at all times, no matter the circumstances
- We work hard
- Do the right thing, for the right reason, all the time
- We are a team of grace

These principles were manifested through hard work, through the constant effort of embracing a growth mindset, through choosing ownership of emotions and attitudes, through seeing circumstances as temporary and finite opportunities, through valuing relationship as the most important element of life, through embracing influence through actions, and through pure effort derived from a motive to a serve beyond one's own ambition. These key principles are the foundation of Messiah Women's Soccer. Many have implications that spilled over into my pursuit towards being a successful leader in life long after my status as a college athlete. A career at Messiah, and being a National Champion, meant more than being skilled at the game of soccer. It was about learning to lead through the principles that defined the culture at MWS. "After all, leaders aren't born, they are made. And they are made just like anything else, through hard work. And that's the price we'll have to pay to achieve that goal, or any goal" (Olson, 2011, p. 88).

My four year journey at Messiah was the most rewarding, most developmental, and the most challenging. I was extremely blessed to have the opportunity to play soccer for such a high achieving institution. I was that one freshman who was "the chance"; the one that may or may not actually see the field. I was the "hopeful". I had the work ethic, the drive, the teachable mindset, the character that Coach was looking for in a recruit. But I wasn't the most technical, tactical, or fast player. And I was short. Still am. But my five foot tall nothing frame was strong and agile. To this day, I am still strong and agile, but my soccer ability has regressed. But at that time, I was determined to use the abilities that I did possess to prove that I was at Messiah for a reason. I was going to have to fight and scrape and prove to Coach that I was worth putting on the game field. I was extremely blessed to represent Messiah, and I wore the #7 jersey with pride. My ultimate desire was to be worthy not only of the name written across my chest, but also continue the legacy of those before me who touted #7. No excuse was going to get in my way.

    I worked incredibly hard through every phase of each year. In-season, post-season, winter training season, spring season, and summer. I put in so many miles on the treadmill, track, back roads, vacation locations - early in the morning, late at night, in gnarly conditions, in old running shoes and ragged cutoff shirts. I wanted to prove myself worthy. My freshman year was a constant struggle to meet and to surpass the current standards of fitness. Beyond freshman year, I wanted to continue to set the standard, across various disciplines that mattered more to the culture than fitness. I desired my conduct, my actions, my integrity, my behavior when I was certain no one cared or was watching, and my attitude to reflect excellence. That was what it was going to take, and excellence drove the key principles I lived by. Excellence drove the philosophy of MWS. Excellence defined at Messiah: "Deliberate actions, ordinary in themselves, performed consistently and correctly, compounded together, added up over time" [Current Messiah Women's Soccer Training Packet]. This reflects Aristotle "We are what we repeatedly do. Excellence, then is not an act but a habit" (Zigarelli, 2011, p. 191). A key element of success and pursuit of excellence returns to the lack of recognition for small and insignificant choices. "We hope to win, but we focus on striving for excellence, which is more under our control than winning" (Zigarelli, 2011, p. 18). We set our sights every year on a National Championship, but we trained every day and made small choices to continually improve. We sought perfection from ourselves every day, not only on the training field, but in every aspect of life. "We strive for perfection even though it's never going to happen in soccer. The closer we get, the better we are" [Scott Frey] (Zigarelli, 2011, p. 185). In all of my pursuits and choice of investments, I was resolved to be uncompromising in my pursuit of perfection, knowing full well I was never going to get there. I was steadfast in my resolve to make small choices that would cause me to step just a little bit closer towards the unattainable goal. I knew that these small choices were not meant for anyone to acknowledge. "At the time you make the simple choices, nobody notices but you. The result at the time of the choice was invisible"(Olson, 2011, p. 38).

    There were always going to be excuses. There was always going to be a reason, a "justification" to be less than excellent. To shortchange a workout. To sleep in. To stay out a little late. To be selfish. To take the work I had accomplished and claim it as my own. To claim that my challenges were more difficult to overcome than my teammates' personal challenges. To view playing time as my motivation and reward. The result of the choices I faced from day to day, compounded year to year, were dependent upon what I believed about myself.

Messiah Women's Soccer symbolized a beautiful struggle. My competitive nature and desire to push myself for the highest of standards were challenged every day. This caused a meaningful and conscious pursuit of excellence. My passionate pursuit of excellence was necessary, if I claimed to truly care about upholding the culture of MWS. Messiah Women's Soccer challenged my very identity. "Giving one's best at all times is a lifestyle, a tradition, 'the dogged pursuit of excellence', and it touches everything from our work ethic to fitness to technical skills to soccer IQ to character to relationships to academics. Playing to standard - and in our case, living to standard- means doing everything with utmost quality and distinction" (Zigarelli, 2011, p. 191). That was, and still is, the way of MWS. I didn't get the playing time that I believed I deserved. I did not receive the accolades that fit the hard work that I invested. I wasn't the iconic top goal scorer who people associated with Messiah's year to year greatness. But the expectations of being a Messiah Women's Soccer player consistently required of me one thing: humbly embrace excellence as a servant leader.

My motivation, as a manifestation of my identity, had to come from a place that was not dependent upon circumstances. It had to come from a place that was not shaken, rocked, or fluctuated due to circumstances or hasty emotional responses. Early in my athletic career at Messiah, despite winning the National Championship in 2011 and in 2012, I questioned my status there. I questioned if I was meant to be there. I questioned if I was valued, as a player and as a person. I was faced with a choice. I wrestled with my "why". Was I going to allow my value to be determined by something that was quantified athletically? By the attention of fans? By my picture on the Messiah athletics web page? By playing time? I had to choose to be validated within my various roles - player, a leader, a teammate - from a constant condition of identity. Not a position.

I oriented my potential to influence towards hard work and humility. This orientation allowed me to pursue excellence with no dependency upon circumstances, and with a confidence of my worth. "Leadership is not a title, but an attitude ... With the standard- bearer concept in place, everyone matters. Everyone is affirmed as having a gift and an essential role. Consequently, players keep buying- in and keep working hard, no matter where they fall on the depth chart" (Zigarelli, 2011, p. 133). To be a standard bearer, I realized that personal expectations had no position in my "how" or in my "why".

I had to choose to deny the expectation of worth based upon athletic achievement.

This process was exactly that - a growing process. I had to wake up and decide each day what I believed about myself, and why what I did was an extension of what I believed. I went through a season of doubt. I battled myself, and how I quantified my worth. Believe me, choosing to embrace excellence was a daily struggle. I remember countless days when I faked being "ok". When I trained my butt off, then trained more on my own after the organized training session ended; when I invested time into my teammates, even when

I wasn't sure if I was meant to be on the team; when I questioned if any of my work would ever pay off... I wondered if I mattered at all. I wondered if my role had any significance. I wondered if I meant anything at all. I realized, by valuing the pursuit of excellence, that my ego and my expectations had no place on this team. Making my TEAM better; making MYSELF a better leader and influence, and cultivating a CULTURE of playing to a standard based upon an identity firmly rooted in hope and love became my attitude orientation. My condition was my choice. My position was out of my control. I didn't always feel like being rooted in hope, love, or joy, and sometimes I had to pretend as though I did. But, I realized that when I allowed my personal agendas [expectations] to become more important than my team and the overarching mission's success, performance suffered and failure was more likely. This concept is reinforced in "_Extreme Ownership_" (Willink & Babin, 2015).

I was able to step into a leadership role that was characterized by joy, by perspective, by hope, by discipline and consistency, by the release of control over an unknown future, by ownership and responsibility of my actions and therefore my teammates' actions, and by doing the hard things. "If 'play to a standard' means anything, it means the the leader will be raising the bar - permanently- insisting on maximum effort, calling out non-adherents, quashing mediocrity, and unswervingly enforcing new thresholds of behavior" (Zigarelli, 2011, p. 207). As I strove for playing to a standard, I operated increasingly from the perspective of a leader. I saw myself as an influence, my actions above reproach. I determined that my foundation, my choice of condition, was to be a consistent place from which I drove my attitude. This mindset became a habit, as my small and seemingly mundane choices compounded day after day, year after year. I had to practice my attitude. I had to reinforce my foundation, through repetition.

There are too many memories from my time at Messiah to describe in sufficient detail. The Commonwealth Championships, NCAA tournaments, and National Championships all highlighted the athletic caliber of MWS. But my time at Messiah was not defined by these achievements. No, I gained much more from Messiah than a few rings and hardware (although they are super cool).

I gained relationships and life lessons that mean more than any NCAA title.

I gained the most fulfilling experiences, the most fun adventures, and the most meaningful memories with my best friends.

Every year, my teammates and I skipped class to watch the NCAA bracket release and review Messiah's position in the standings. We were like little kids, giddy with excitement as we looked what other teams were on "our side" of the bracket, and which teams appeared to have the best records. We anticipated the late fall with anxiety and excitement; we were giddy. NCAA season was what we trained for all year. The tournament was why we cared so much about pursuing excellence since the beginning of the post-season the year prior. Each and every practice and game mattered if we hoped to reach the NCAA tournament. It all mattered. And NCAA season mattered most. We had to take care of business in the regular season competitions to be able to establish our place in the bracket. We had to take care of each game as if it were our last. I remember Coach reminding us of the value of each game. He said "Next game, last game", to indicate that to have a last game, we need to take care of the next game. And we wanted the last game of the season to be a National Championship game. Each game mattered. Each game was one more chance to compete with my sisters. Each game was a stepping stone towards the last game.

Fall was the BEST time of year. Teammates who had similar majors would choose class schedules based on how many of us could be in the same classes. MWS had a "special" table in the dining hall. When walking around campus, we traveled as a posse. We laughed at and with each other, wherever we went. We created fun out of everything. We were easy to spot out on campus, repping our MWS gear, 3/4 pants, fun socks, and of course, outrageous tan lines. Walks to and from the practice field were loud and obnoxious as we got out the "gigs" before having to dial in for the training set. No matter what, MWS was a team; and we loved each other just as fiercely as we competed.

Throughout my MWS career, I gained perspective; I gained identity forged through the flames of trial. I was stripped of what I had previously thought had defined me. I gained the ability to put my own desires aside, and labor for a purpose greater than myself. I gained relationships that will last a lifetime; I gained the beauty of appreciating every teammate around me as an essential part of the culture of MWS. I gained truth and understanding regarding discipline, consistency, and the power of habit. I gained the value of taking ownership. I learned that love and servanthood are necessary for success as an individual, and as a team. I learned and practiced the tools necessary to become a leader. As described in the _"The Messiah Method"_, being a standard bearer was the way to reveal your position as a member of MWS. "Do your best at everything, but be great at something that matters to the team. Model it for your teammates. Raise the bar for everyone. Take on a role. Be a standard bearer "(Zigarelli, 2011, p. 132).

MWS is more than a soccer program with one of the most winningest coaches in NCAA history. MWS is more than an a four year college experience. MWS is a special culture; it utilizes faith and sport and selfless love to develop leaders. It utilizes tangible outcomes of soccer and seamlessly integrates development of character as the ultimate result. It can only be fully understood by those who have contributed, sacrificed, and fought to maintain and to enhance the culture of excellence. My experience at Messiah was an athletic venture defined by relationships and love. Further, my experiences were forged through development of character by means of the power choice. It was defined by the effort of relationships. Love expressed through servant leadership and purpose expressed through genuine care defined my journey.

MWS will forever hold special place in my heart. It will forever be a place in which I look back confidently that my time there was maximized. I have no regrets. I smile contentedly as I reminisce the investment of hard work, choices, mentality, faith and trust, and the beautiful relationships that so richly filled my heart during my career.

The experiences and the development I received as an athlete and as a person at Messiah have caused me to step into life with a confidence and high sense of self awareness. Little did I know that the leadership and character principles that I learned as an athlete are integral to leadership and to success on a broad scale. These principles are effective tactics towards development within other team atmospheres. There are dichotomies that exist within the Messiah Women's Soccer culture; and some of these dichotomies are present within the structure of the Navy Seals. Dichotomies woven into training and play, into culture, and into the consistency of MWS are:

    Fiercely competitive spirit AND selfless love
    Hardest working team AND most technical team
    Champion's heart AND humble spirit
    Driven individuals AND selfless teammates
    Dare greatly AND the courage to fail
    GOAL: to be a champion AND being a champion is not our purpose
    (Zigarelli, 2011, p. 89).

These seemingly opposing ideas are consciously practiced every single day at Messiah. These dichotomies are not singular to my experiences as an NCAA athlete. Successful leaders in SEAL teams require these characteristics, among others:

        Aggressive BUT not overbearing
        A leader must be calm BUT not robotic
        A leader must be confident BUT never cocky
        A leader must be brave BUT not foolhardy
        Competitive BUT a gracious loser
        Attentive to details BUT not obsessed by them
        Strong BUT have endurance
        A leader AND follower
        Humble BUT not passive
        Aggressive BUT not overbearing
        Quiet BUT not silent
        Logical BUT not devoid of emotions

(Willink & Babin, 2015).

The opposing qualities practiced by leaders are delicate to balance; requiring time, energy, and toughness to become habitual. The presence of conflicting qualities integrated in the Messiah culture, "the genius of the AND", is similar to the presence of the conflicting themes of other leaders. Leaders must dedicate effort and attention to these conflicting qualities, while practicing effective communication.

Effort and sacrifice in order to balance and demonstrate these dichotomies are what successful leaders do.

Within any team, a leader takes responsibility. A leader steps up. A leader takes ownership. A leader is humble. A leader seeks the needs of others before their own. A leader serves without expectation of acknowledgement. A leader listens. A leader is an example by word and deed. A leader is made. "Leadership is not something you "do", it is something that grows organically out of the natural rhythm of learning"(Olson, 2011, p. 154).

The more I desired to learn how to be a better leader, and how to integrate the "genius of the AND" into my habits and my identity, the reality of my ability to lead was actualized. As I pursued learning, I gained an ability to communicate more effectively, and thus I gained an ability to teach. "Great leaders must be great teachers. Otherwise, few are influenced. Few follow. Skeptical? See how many you can name who are one but not the other" (Zigarelli, 2011, p. 150). Effective communication and careful listening skills are trademarks of teachers. Teachers lead. Choosing to learn, choosing to grow, choosing to seek something greater than yourself is where leadership, success, and winning begin.

Now, we will begin to identify how to Execute.
Get ready.

CHAPTER 2

DO THINGS

 Another mile. Another hot, lonely, dreaded mile. Waking up at the (butt)crack of dawn to run the first timed mile of the summer (alone) was how every June began. Summer training for Messiah Women's Soccer included track workouts; the pace of which were determined by timed mile trials. Timed miles were spaced intermittently through the summer, based upon the weekly schedule of training in the summer workout packet. And each one caused equally as much anxiety as the one prior. Each time you ran the mile, you were responsible for tracking your result, which you could share with Coach or with the team. Your mile time dictated your pace for training during the summer months. The timed mile was a fitness test of preseason. Six minutes was the standard. If you could run a six minute mile at the beginning of the summer, the expectation was to run it faster. My first ever timed mile at the beginning of June before my freshman year was 6:14. My preseason mile time test result was a 6:03. I had improved over the summer. And I had made myself better. Eventually, I was able to run my best mile time, a 5:40. The point was to raise the standard for yourself.

 Raising the standard on a personal level caused us to be better as a team, raising the standard was the culture.

Running, soccer specific workouts with a ball, speed and agility training, and strength training were components of the summer training workout packet. Each day was planned, and the weekly schedule was identical for each player during the summer. The expectation was for each player to come into the season personally fit and ready to meet demands of the highest level of NCAA DIII soccer. There was no ceiling to fitness. No matter how fit a player was, they were charged to become more fit. No matter how technically sound a player was, they were expected to refine their touch even more. No matter what the fitness starting point was at the beginning of the summer, the expectation was to become better. Every day offered the choice to do the work- and not just performing it to get it off the list- but setting it as the priority. The mindset being: "I will become better at the completion of this workout. I will give it my all." It was hard to train with this intensity, and to train "all out" when I had no teammates around me to train with.

I completed the summer training packet on my lonesome. Lonely training served as yet another tool of internal development and character.

I lived in rural Pennsylvania, not close enough to any of my teammates to train with them. I trained every day, alone. I used a high school track to run, the stadium turf to train, and the back country roads (cross country routes I used to run in high school) to be my terrain to prepare for season and to complete each day of training. When not around my normal stomping grounds, I would scope out patches of grass, hills, 1/2 mile stretches of road/beach/flat surface, parks or swing sets, in order to train daily. I would wake up early on vacation to do my speed and agility on the beach; or to do interval sprints in the hotel parking lot; or to run paced track-style workouts on a flat (enough) surfaces.

The summer packet offered a guide; a schedule. Did I HAVE to follow it? Nope. Did anyone check in and make sure I did the workout for the day? Sometimes. Was anyone going to know if I "cheated" a workout by a few reps? Nope. I had choices every day. I had to choose to show up. I had to choose to invest in the workout. I had to choose to prioritize it, even on vacation (no matter where I was), to get up early to avoid the summer sun. The choice before me every day was to ignore the circumstances of life around me in order to pursue preparation. The goal that drove the preparation was a national championship- the pinnacle of NCAA athletic pursuits. The extremely high value of the goal caused the expectations of preparation to be set equally as high, equally as worthy of the goal. "Coach set high expectations, he enforced high expectations"(Zigarelli, 2011, p. 197).

Each summer, I had the same choices to make. My ability to influence and the weight of leadership that I carried increased with my maturity from year to year. I grew more into a leader on the team, and thus, more was expected of me from season to season. If the "dogged pursuit of excellence" as a student athlete wasn't consuming enough, I was being stretched personally at home. Behind the scenes I was emotionally struggling with my parents' divorce. I was processing my own emotional responses while at the same time trying to shield my younger sister from the negative relational strain. I worked various summer jobs (one was working a glorious first shift at Dunkin Donuts, another was shoveling horse manure), and altering my workout times between morning and evening made my daily schedule absolute chaos. I worked so hard to be a sister, a friend, a daughter, a "mom" role of my family at home, confidant to perplexed family members, a teammate, and the most prepared player for MWS. I felt as though I was always shifting my mental and emotional and physical aura to be the biggest impact for those around me. But these were all circumstances. No excuse could justify a lack of effort. No reason was acceptable to pursue excellence any less passionately than when life was easier. I owned and processed my trials without telling my teammates. There was no way I could succumb to hardships, and expect sympathy. There was no way I was giving in. To be "soft" disgusts me. And I would not allow my struggles to overflow into my ability to train. I would not and could not allow lack of sleep, fatigue, relational strain, and life responsibilities to be "reasons" not to lead, or train with all out abandon. No one knew. And I wasn't going to tell them. I had to suck it up. I had to value something over the circumstances. And I did. I expected myself to prove it.

The long, hard, lonely summers between freshman year and senior year were periods of incredible personal development. And it was all up to me. My aspiration was to deny excuses. There could be no reason valid for me to be "standard". I had many reasons- justifications- to not work so hard. My broken family, the challenge of leadership, the time invested to relationships and the responsibility of having several jobs… all valid reasons to be content with average. Yet. That is not excellence. That is not leadership. "Leaders require courage. Change provokes resistance and overcoming resilience requires courage. Bold leadership. A willingness to stand firm in the face of those vested in the status quo" (Zigarelli, 2011, p. 206). Status quo? Gross.

Everything that I was taught; everything that I was learning through MWS revolved around the pursuit of excellence. Doing the small, mundane, and seemingly unimportant acts in and of themselves on a consistent basis was something I was in complete control of. My emotions were always my choice. My attitudes and my behavior were always my responsibility.

We all possess reasons or excuses to remain content; but we all have have the ability to seize ownership. I would not let myself be anything less than that of what I knew to be possible. What was possible? Being better. What was achievable was in my hands. I had to risk; I had to see failure as opportunity. I had to seize each day and each workout. I had to become comfortable with the idea of failure. I had to understand that failure was necessary to succeed. If I had chosen to be sure of the outcome of each day, I never would have grown. If I had chosen to remain comfortable, I would have no power to influence. I had high expectations for myself; I would be the role model, the leader, the influence that I needed to be through my due diligence. What did that require? Doing things, the small things, practiced over and over. My thoughts and my attitudes meant nothing until an action followed. The action that followed either propelled me one step closer in the pursuit of excellence, or it revealed a weakness in my ability to own my choices.

Summer workouts never became any easier, because the thought process was to always push yourself as hard as possible. But consistency made the choice to get up early, to embrace burning lungs, to welcome sore and tired legs, to schedule intermittent naps, and to lead through actions not seen by anyone became easier. Doing things, based upon my choice of attitude and my identity, through hard work were contributions and standards for the team. I prioritized the goal of a National Championship, which had to be revealed by my pursuit of fitness. I prioritized the chemistry of my team, which had to be revealed by my steadfast resolve to deny comfort zones. Energy fueled by my prioritization of preparation resulted in accomplishment of the little things. To perform things that were tough; to inspire others and reveal to them that mental toughness and resilience is key in the pursuit of success.

To embrace a realistic goal that required personal and individual effort were actions that I did in order to validate and prove my mindset as a leader.

Why was doing things important? For the pursuit of a greater goal. A goal means nothing without action. Action means doing. No one else can pursue your goal for you. Even if the goal is something that is intangible; such as becoming a better leader.

How you do become a better leader? Practice it. "In order to become a leader and to build a team that performs at the highest levels, leadership qualities must be enhanced through practice and through training. How do you practice? Start with looking in the mirror. Check the ego. Take responsibility for mistakes, expectations, effort, and priorities" (Willink & Babin, 2015).

What do you prioritize?
Where do you spend your time, energy, and money?
It is there where your priority is; no matter what you claim with your words. Your actions through your investments clearly reveal your priorities.

Whatever you prioritize, why do you prioritize it?

If your time, energy, and money are being spent in ways that are not aligning with what you *claim* priorities are, then re-evaluate your fears and your ego. Re-establish the true, authentic, desires of your heart. Strip away priorities that are not your own. Align your actions with the truth of priorities.

Do you really value health? Or do you actually just value a "perfect" body?

Do you value the cohesion of your family? Or you do you actually value how you believe people perceive your role within your family unit?

Take and honest moment to check your pride, your priorities, and your actions.

"Intentionality and attention to detail are touchstones of success. Leaders invest heavily in the routines; striving to create an environment where execution is more likely. To win, you have to execute. Execution requires readiness. Readiness is no accident. At Messiah, it happens through purposeful, road tested processes" (Zigarelli, 2011, p. 83). Processes require action, through thoughtful preparation, and repetition. Habits are created and purpose is revealed through practice. Practice indicates growth of skills necessary to engrain a habit into the process, becoming more effective, systematically, over time."Practice communicating effectively, by listening and choosing a response permeated in humility. Practice viewing circumstances as opportunities for growth. Practice being calm and consistent despite chaos. Practice being a servant and being an encourager to those around you. How do you become a leader? Expect little from others; demand the best from yourself" (Willink & Babin, 2015).

Do things.

CHAPTER 3

FELT COUCHES

    My grandpa owned a cabin in upstate Pennsylvania, located in a remote area almost completely off the grid. My grandpa frequented the cabin less as he got older, and my family was able to utilize it more. Rocky and rugged mountains surround the cabin on all sides. Networks of trails throughout the mountains offered opportunity to see deer, turkeys, and bears in their natural habitat. The Pine Creek flowed essentially through the front yard of the cabin, and allowed plenty of opportunity for kayak launches, canoe excursions, and tubing adventures. An old railroad bed near the cabin was converted to a Rail Trail, and allowed miles of biking, running, and walking. Although the seasons of the year each offered beauty, adventure, and peace from the noise of civilization, the fall was especially beautiful and incredibly special. The fall season included crisp morning air, outdoor solitude, and best of all, vibrant colors of leaf changes. The prettiest of reds and maroons; various shades of orange and yellow, and tones of green conifers that painted the sidehills made each fall season simply beautiful.

    The cabin has been a work in progress, in terms of physical structure. When the cabin was passed on to my family, my dad had a choice: torch it to the ground - it was in really bad shape - or restore the original structure from the foundation up. Dad decided to take on the latter project. The magnitude of stripping down the cabin to its bare bones and re-establishing its structure resulted in work-oriented cabin trips. My family would tow a camper behind the pickup truck and live from the camper as we worked to make the cabin actually suitable for living. Dad was methodical about how he went about bringing life back into the cabin - the cinder block foundation, supporting beams of the floor, floorboards, ceiling supports, rafters, ties, and ridge beams… then an addition built from the dirt up….to complete the shape of the cabin. Each trip to the cabin always included some sort of accomplishment. Little details were accomplished, each one contributing towards restoration.

After years of work, the physical structure was restored, and the cabin was (fairly) livable. But, the interior had yet to be addressed. The cabin had not had any furniture or kitchen or bathroom updates in decades. The stale, moldy, and fusty odor of the cabin was the most easily recognizable trait to indicate that some updating was indeed necessary. Or at least febreeze plugins, candles, or wax melters. Other interior characteristics that needed addressing were yellow glowing light fixtures, sulfur stained sinks and toilets, shag rugs, a plastic sofa (for real, it still exists), and a felt couch. This felt couch was detailed with mustard yellow and baby blue flowers (now being more like a faded brownish gold and faded gray slate blue-ish). That couch has been in the cabin ever since my earliest memories of the cabin - and to this day, it is not only still in existence, but it is my dad's favorite couch. Should anything happen to that couch, dad would not only be quite upset, but would also no longer have his most comfortable place. That couch is dad's favorite place to rest and breathe a deep satisfied sigh after a long hard day's work.

    The cabin transformation took many years. It took lots of planning and preparation. To strip it down and start basically from scratch took so much time and effort for my parents, and for me and my siblings. As much as we loved the cabin for adventuring, campfires, and clowning around, we were always expected to work on the projects that dad tasked us with. Hauling cinder blocks, mixing concrete, chopping logs for firewood, carrying supplies to certain areas of construction, stripping siding, staining boards, digging drainage ditches, clawing away old insulation….the cabin transformation process was hard work. Yet, I never viewed a trip to the cabin as "work". In fact, some of my most fond of memories are from those "work" trips. It was *always* fun to exert hard work and concentrated energy, with the expectation of what was to come. The expectation of a comfortable cabin in the future made the effort always worth it. Phase after phase, year after year, working on the cabin was a dynamic process. Each trip to the cabin included fun activities that utilized the natural environment. We made it a priority to take full advantage of what the outdoors freely offered! Furthermore, the changes around the cabin as the construction phases morphed from one to another offered new forms of fun. For example, assembling the addition required setting up and framing the foundation. The cinder block foundation was laid, and it served as a perimeter to surround a perfect rectangle of soft, silty dirt within its border. This dirt space was to eventually be covered by concrete and floorboards. But until that phase of construction, the cinder blocks restrained the silty dirt area. The soil had no rocks in it, and when it got wet, it became a natural slip and slide. Slippery and sloppy dirt sounded like a perfect venue for fun. My siblings and I could not let an opportunity such as this slip us by. Pun intended. We decided to make a dirt "race track" within this interior rectangle, the cinder blocks being the perimeter. We established a serpentine track with simply our bare feet, running lap after lap, easily beating down a clear course. Once the course was easily recognized in dry conditions, we added a little water, and lo and behold, the Indy-500 Slip and Slide Footrace was born. My siblings and I literally raced around that track, slipping and sliding and falling and covering ourselves in mud - for hours. I cannot even attempt to venture how many miles we ran, with no concept of being "tired" or counting the laps or determining how far we ran. We just ran. The more we ran, the more fun we had. The more fun we had, the more we ran. I don't think anyone could have had as much fun as we did with just a little dirt, water, and bare feet.

 The cabin went through a major transformation to become the vacation home, the comfort space, the place of respite and peace that it is today. It is an escape from civilization and from "normal". Years of effort, time, sweat, and finances were spent on its behalf. And now we reap the benefits of relaxation, a fulfilling and unquantifiable reward for the sacrifices. The sacrifices given were worth every moment, every penny, every momentary discomfort. Dad had a vision for the cabin, and only now are we able to experience the reality of Dad's vision. However, the process of bringing that vision to life is what has made the cabin so much more than a structure. The hard work we put into that architecture; the tedious, seemingly endless, and monotonous steps that were required to prepare for another work weekend; the lessons learned putting in work before "play", were all part of the cabin process. The re-creation of the cabin resulted not in simply a place; it created character.

The cabin was dirty. It was stinky. It was old. The water was gross. There was no cellular service (when I was a kid, wifi wasn't a thing yet, and of course there was none of that. Plus, there was no need for it. You don't need wifi to hike and to kayak and to lay cinder blocks and to dig ditches...) The closest Walmart or Target was 45 minutes away. The cabin wasn't always "pleasant". But that is what made it special.

The greater vision of what the cabin could be caused the circumstances to seem less unpleasant. I do not remember the "unpleasant" as much as I remember the enjoyments and the amusements. I remember the time spent with my family, working towards a common goal; and enjoying the small things along the way (like slip and slides, the creek, and the campfires). The work was hard. The fun was real. And the cabin holds the experiences of my character development within its very walls and foundation.

The cabin is a symbol of a growth process. A mindset of growth allows one to seize momentary choices as opportunities. An attitude of growth alters a perspective, incorporating personal ownership to position one's self progressively closer towards a goal. Some goals take a modest progression, occurring over years and years. Other goals can be quickly actualized. What matters most is the buy in- the commitment- towards growing in the hope of something greater. Goal setting is essential for every leader; it governs the direction of effort. As I learned at Messiah through the wisdom of Coach Frey, "the only thing worse than running is not having something to run for" (Zigarelli,

2011, p. 24). I ran and trained with a goal of fitness and increased athletic performance. My conditioning and intentional training habits revealed my ability to lead through goal orientation and ensuing action. A leader must assess and set a goal for themselves, and for their team. The realistic process to attain that goal must also be evaluated. However, if a leader does not establish a systematic structure to attain the goal, then it is simply an idea. It's easy to have a goal, a nice idea, an imagined reality. We all have them. We all have dreams. That which separates those that succeed and those that fail is the commitment to growth. The adoption of a growth mindset. It's an attitude; a viewpoint, that dictates the actions taken to bring the goal to fruition. It's a choice to see circumstances as opportunities; it's a choice to make decisions and identify priorities that will advance you closer to your goal. Viewing a challenge as an opportunity, as a chance to be seized, is a trademark mindset of successful leaders. How much you value the goal is reflected by how you commit to and value each step of the process. Committing to the process is expressed and manifested through action. The cabin was once uninhabitable. It has become a place of peace, restoration, and contentment, but only through a long and arduous process.

You too can transition and transform your current position. You can begin your process at any time. "It is important to start on the path and to remember that no matter what has gone on before, you can begin fresh and new, and at any time you can choose to start with a clean slate " (Olson, 2011, p.53). It may be hard to quantify the value of setting the goal and planning the process. However, the lack of quantification causes the commitment to be priceless. Quantification indicates a ceiling of reward; the value of discipline, habit, and commitment can be pursued with an excitement of limitless reward.

Vocalizing a goal can create an image of actuality. But until action is taken, until disciplined choices are made consistently, until responsibility is taken for the actions taken toward the undertaking, the goal is as real as seeing the wind. Seize your process. No one else can. Blame no circumstances (or smelly odors, or sulfur stained toilet bowls); we all have excuses.

But you can decide. Your process is up to you. Circumstances are in flux; and circumstances do not determine your path. Do not believe in the fallacy that your path forward is dictated by circumstances.

As you embrace the process, smile. Have fun. It'll be a journey; with victories and challenges and circumstances of various forms. But each experience offers an opportunity to grow you in knowledge and in influence. There is a little risk involved. There is fear too. There are things beyond your control. How much do you value the goal? Embrace the process, each little step at a time. The unpredictability is what makes the journey that much more special. The chance to pursue an unquantifiable reward is where influence is waiting to be seized. Do not allow it to pass you by. Once the chance is gone, it cannot return. Commit to the process. And have fun along the way. The moments along your process and your path make it unique and special and only determined by you.

If you need a moment to rest on this journey, there is a faded felt yellow couch withstanding the test of time that offers the best nap venue.

CHAPTER 4

ALL THE COFFEE, SOCIAL WEDNESDAYS, DUCKLINGS

As a sports medicine professional and a strength and conditioning coach, I have been trained in nutrition, physiology, biological adaptations, and other physical processes that influence performance. However, my experiences in grad school caused me to question my own academic training. Could I survive off of exercise, coffee, popcorn, wine, and 4 hours of sleep for two years? Is there enough coffee in this universe to support my excessive intake? If a body that is in motion remains in motion, is sleep necessary (riddle me that, Sir Isaac Newton)?

Pursuing a masters degree in sports medicine research at the University of Pittsburgh (Pitt) immediately after my undergraduate education was an incredible opportunity. I wanted to continue to pursue exercise and performance science, yet I wanted to be involved with the emergence of cutting edge research. I wanted to break through previous understandings and solve unanswered questions regarding athletic performance. I was eager to learn and to serve high achieving athletes and military populations at the Neuromuscular Research Laboratory (NMRL) and complete my degree with a thesis. A thesis project required an extensive background, literature review, detailed methodologies, and comprehensive discussion of applications. From data collection methods and rationale, statistical analysis, results, and discussion concerning the relevance of my findings, this project was epitome of my degree. My project purpose was to identify relationships of risk factors surrounding energy available for muscles and the presence of fatigue in female soccer players. Along with learning how to properly conduct research and perform scientific procedures, I learned how to utilize a novel method using ultrasound technology to assess muscular fuel levels. To validate my data collection methods, my advisor and I ran an independent study to precede my actual thesis pursuit.

There were two other classmates at Pitt who ventured to pursue a thesis along with me. These two girls were also my roommates, Jordan and Alice. Our other classmates opted to complete their degree via a scholarly research paper. This option was available to those who were not as interested in the research process. Jordan and Alice and I lived together, did school together, and collectively decreased the global coffee bean availability by a large percentage. All three of us worked long hours at our respective jobs, while pursuing our degrees and coursework at the NMRL, and exerted extra effort to formulate our thesi (our term to describe multiple thesis projects).

The three of us were aided in the pursuit of our degrees by a PhD student at the NMRL, who at any given point in time would drop everything to help us. Her name is Anne. But we knew her as Momma Duck. She guided us through the meticulous world of the data collection processes. She simplified the research world so that we could entertain the hope of thesi completion and graduation. Without her help, graduation was imaginary. As Anne was constructing her dissertation, teaching classes, and working on other projects at the lab, she still put aside time and energy to lead her "ducklings" on the path to success….oh, and she was also planning her wedding. Momma Duck- Anne -was essential to the completion of my thesis and graduation. I owe her an enormous amount of gratitude, and the highest quality of coffee beans. Jordan and Alice and I worked our butts off in grad school, often comparing stories of our diverse work experiences, and sharing frustrations over the arduous and (quite frankly) aggravating research process. After a long day of both sciencing and working, Jordan and I would convalesce in the kitchen and catch up about our day as we completed our biostatistics homework. We would usually be looking at one problem for hours… until Alice would get home from work. Alice worked ridiculously long hours, and would get home super late. Alice would barely have crossed the threshold of the doorway before Jordan and I would woefully ask for help. Alice, without complaint, would show us the answer within seconds of looking at the problem. If the problem was REALLY tough, it would take Alice a minute or two to figure it out and explain the solution. No matter how little sleep she had, she would graciously aid Jordan and I. Alice too would convalesce with us, as we continued with sharing experiences of the day as we completed the homework together, and then retire (collapse) from exhaustion.

During grad school, I worked as a personal trainer, and my hours typically began at 5am. My last clients of the day sometimes concluded at 10pm. I was also an actively competing Spartan athlete and trail ultramarathoner; my days were a blur of science, coaching my clients, and pursuing my own athletic endeavors. Among Jordan, Alice, and I, we didn't have much social time, nor the finances to participate in many social events. However, we made time to prioritize our collective presence at a bar called Social. Social was within walkable distance of home. Social was *our* place. The bartenders knew us by name, knew about science endeavors (based solely on hearing our collective complaints), knew how to make us laugh, knew what sports we wanted to watch, knew our drink choices....we were regulars. Social offered drink specials on Wednesdays. These specials advertised specific cans of beer being just a mere $2 or $3. Being in a social environment with cheap beers appealed greatly to us Ducklings. Wednesday nights at Social were our nights. When we were at Social, we beefed up our collective title of "Ducklings". We referred to ourselves as "Battle Buddies". This title gave us rationale behind the bags under our eyes, and justified our intense outbursts regarding our research projects. Going to Social on Wednesdays allowed us just a few hours to be normal humans. We relished the rare chance to relax over a beer or two, to watch a sporting event, and to share friendship over shared appetizers. Wednesdays at Social allowed us the chance to release a little stress, and to be *almost* regular people.

There was a consistent theme throughout my grad school experience that aided survival - sarcasm. It was the only way to withstand the ultimate confusion of each day, each obstacle, each challenge that confounded us. Lectures, projects, setbacks, difficult relationships and conflicts with significant others, bitter cold Pittsburgh winters, and other perturbations to any shred of normalcy was met with a phrase.

"It's fine."

Which was followed immediately by another phrase.

"It's always fine."

Truth be told, it was *anything* but fine. It was quite the opposite; but, if we vocalized and laughed (through very real tears), about being "fine", somehow, someway, it became "fine." Focus, determination, grit, encouragement and advice, and prioritization were components of our personal lives that caused our struggles to eventually become just fine. But until we knew how to make it fine, we used the phrase as a bluff, to minimize the giant mountains of adversity that we faced.

"It's fine" was said more and more often as circumstances seemed insurmountable, however, the hope of what we were striving for caused us to conclude that "it's fine" no matter what. It had to be. There was no option for it to be otherwise.

Our belief in "it's fine" reflected our growth mindset- to strive to position ourselves in a way that would actualize being "fine". That is how we progressed. That is how we moved forward. We had to believe that a future reality was real, while living in a different reality at the present. If I believed truly that "it's fine" and that I can succeed through my struggles, then my behavior would echo that mindset. Things weren't really "fine", but I trusted that, through hard work, discipline, choices of priorities, that things could be "fine". By believing in the actualization of that future reality, I was able to step forward and bring that reality to fruition.

On the flipside, if I chose to believe that my circumstances were insurmountable, then I denied hope. I could have denied a growth mindset, and settled into a stagnant and complacent state in which "fine" would never be attained. It would be just a fleeting condition. With the presence of my roommates, friends, family, and coffee (and running, wine, and the occasional tequila)... "it's fine" became real.

It is incredibly hard to live towards a purpose, or to a future meaning, that is not a current actualization. Believing that a future reality is attainable and understanding that we alone are responsible for its materialization are both necessary. "Meaning must be fulfilled by the man alone; only then does it achieve a significance which will satisfy his own will to meaning" (Frankl, 2006, p. 99).

Simply, stepping into your purpose, your meaning, may require you to fake it a little until you make it. This does not negate or minimize the struggles along the way. Forging ahead towards something that is not yet realized is a risky venture. There is no distinct path ahead, and there is no guarantee of the future.

But when is there ever an absolute guarantee of future events anyway?

The mindset that drives behavior towards a future reality is the character building component that creates momentum once it becomes a habit. Mindset is adopted, and habits result. You choose your thought patterns, and thus, belief. By believing that a future state is attainable, your behavior will reveal the depth of resolve towards this future state. "Man has [both] potentialities within himself; which one is actualized depends on the decisions not on the conditions" (Frankl, 2006, p. 134).

This reality was spoken by one who was in severely limiting conditions; one in which the reality of death was a daily possibility. If he [Frankl] had the hope to voice the belief in the facade "it's fine"; then I am in no way justified in allowing circumstances to determine my position towards potential. Embracing an unknown path forward involves risk. It is scary, and fear is a common emotional choice due to uncertainty. But fear is not justified. The amount of investment you commit to fear, to uncertainty, to unpredictability of the future can cause sidestepping and delays towards the actualization of your purpose or goal.

A brief example of this can be through fitness and health. You may seek a future "state" or goal. You may seek a goal to lose that stubborn 10lbs, or you may be seeking to break a 6 minute mile time. Both of those goals can be future realities. The strength of your belief that they can become realities will determine your next steps: behavior will emulate the belief.

Do you believe that you are capable to achieve a future meaning, future goal?

Decide what is hindering you from a lack of belief. Decide if you value the steps necessary to reach the goal.

Choose to evaluate how greatly a future reality affects your current beliefs.

Determine how much you care about what you cannot currently quantify.

"A weak body will hinder physical performance, but so does a weak mind. For example, consider a pull-up. Most people who lack the belief they all ever do a pull-up, so they never do. As a result, they aren't able to stick with the process long enough to see improvement" (Milner, 2019).

Life pursuits, paths towards success, and fitness all reflect a state of the mind and the power of belief.

"It's fine" was a coping mechanism, but it was linked to a belief. I had to believe that the process of becoming "fine" was attainable. The same goes with health and fitness parameters. Lifestyle changes that support the process of attaining better health and fitness attributes are all within reach. Join a running club; sign up for a race; register for a gym membership; be bold enough to believe. Then continue to act in a way that strengthens and validates that belief. Your goal to improve yourself, to pursue a growth mindset might make other people around you uncomfortable. Their orientation to be comfortable has no bearing over your choices to become uncomfortable. Your choices to embrace discomfort may cause others to become aware of their stagnant state of contentment and comfort. Good. And they may resent you for breaking the mold of contentment. Allow such response to serve as validation for your mindset. Let such a response fuel the courage behind your efforts and pursuits. Circumstances may cause life to be not quite "fine"; but you need to begin the process - in your mind, followed by action - in order to expect any progress towards "fine".

It begins with a choice.

And it begins with coffee.

And a pull-up. Or simply hanging from a bar. Well, maybe coffee isn't exactly a requirement. "Even the weakest among us can develop the strength necessary to do a pull-up" (Milner, 2019).

So pull-ups might actually be a real requirement.

You can develop strength of body, strength of mind. And, you are worth it. There is no room in a mind fixed on growth for fear.

It may not seem or feel like it in the moment, but it can be "fine". Just ask Momma Duck and the Battle Buddies. We will encourage you with shouts of "it's fine"!

It's always fine.

CHAPTER 5

TOUGH

Tough is a quality I learned as a kid. My parents and my older brother were my role models, and I observed their actions to learn what being tough looked like. Tough was a way of life for my family. Toughness was second nature, reflected through mindset and action. Growing up in rural Pennsylvania, most of my time was spent outdoors, working and playing. Being tough meant getting the job done - and most things that needed done required just a little bit of toughness.

Being tough also meant accepting the fact that dirt and maybe some sweat were likely involved in a task.

But dirt doesn't hurt anyone.

And dirt can be fun.

Daily activities, chores, fun, and "Cowboys and Indians" were all accomplished outdoors and included some degree of dirt.

Among fighting with tree branch swords, building numerous forts, creating mountain bike trails, and using our imaginations to create fun, the enjoyments shared with my siblings involved being outdoors. And involved a high risk of injury and pain. And a probability of a visit to the emergency room. But in the name of fun, risk was definitely worth it! It didn't help that we did most of our activities in bare feet. When injuries occurred, there was a general and very simple understanding: if you weren't dying, rub some dirt on it and play on. If the injury was super serious, a band-aid might be an option. But in the rare occurrence that dirt and band-aids were ineffective, mom and dad would take very purposeful actions to seek medicare care.

One of my favorite "tough" activities that my siblings and I enjoyed was only a reality in the winter. A heavy snowfall was all we needed. After a snowfall, we would take off our socks and shoes, wear shorts and T-shirts, and race barefoot laps around the house as many times as we could. The last person to "give in" to cold feet was the winner! Do I remember how cold my feet got? Nope. What I do remember was laughing and sprinting and kicking my feet up as fast as I could, straining with all my might to beat my siblings. I remember circling the house over and over.

I still have all my toes.

Who was toughest of us? Who would ignore frozen feet? Which one of us could withstand the onset of being entirely numb?

Competition was on.

And it was so fun.

I found that wearing T-shirts and shorts in the winter was completely appropriate, when body heat was less important than winning.

Body heat was maintained by the effort of sprinting and by the sheer effort of determination.

I was resolved to win, and being cold wasn't an option!

I didn't always win, but I sure ran as hard as possible.

To this day, my toes and fingers are the first things to get uncomfortably cold, especially on snowboarding trips high into the mountains. Maybe I would stay warm if I ran up the slopes, racing my brother and sister.

Running around the house barefoot in knee high snow and in freezing temperatures was all fun and games. But looking back, I realize that it was a training tool that integrated toughness into who I am. My competitive spirit, and my energy to go all out for the sake of "winning" caused me to set aside the discomfort of freezing feet. I didn't know I was being "tough"; all I knew was that I wanted to beat my siblings.

Winning was my focus.
Being cold was of less importance.

Toughness doesn't mean hiding emotions, covering pain, or ignoring physical, mental, or emotional warning signs. It indicates a perseverance and a resolve, to value an end goal over a temporary distraction or circumstance. It indicates a focus. I firmly and personally believe that being tough matters only in relevance to focus towards the end goal. Pursuing a goal should entail the most efficient way of pursuing that goal. If struggle to persevere is unnecessary in pursuit of the goal, then what are you really trying to prove? If the most efficient way to pursue a goal creates a struggle and a need to persevere, then toughness is a quality that can be developed purposefully. Toughness, at its simplest, is deciding to prioritize something over discomfort. The ability to remain steadfast and embrace toughness over a given period of time, or season, ties into the concept of resilience.

Resilience, by definition, is the "ability to recover from adversity" (Dictionary.com, 2019).

Being resilient is the long haul version of toughness and perseverance. As a child running around in the snow, I was not aware of that environment being a proven venue for the development of resilience. My siblings and I were outside; simply running around like banshees. It was simple enjoyment in nature. All that we needed was snow. Little did we know that we were proof of science. We embraced snow and toughness simultaneously, yet all we knew was that we were having fun. "Nature is a learning resource that promotes resilience in young people and positively affects their future lifecourse opportunities"(Barton, Bragg, Wood, & Pretty, 2016).

In retrospect, my development of resilience was gleaned in the venue of nature.

A resilience mindset is next level. Resilience implies a habit of not giving in when a situation requires endurance and discomfort. It is a permanence of toughness throughout a changing, chaotic, or unpredictable environment. Resilience is a habit, therefore, it must be practiced. The more it is embraced, the more habitual it will become.

As an NCAA athlete, I began to practice resiliency at 18 years old. A freshman on a National Championship team meant that I was expected to work and train and challenge the standard with as much intensity as the sophomores, juniors, and seniors. Freshman year was a learning process, and held no promise of playing time despite the hard work that I did. No matter the number of minutes I accrued on the field, I was expected to train just as hard and with just as much tenacity as the seniors. To work as hard as possible, to sell out every day at training, to concentrate on the details of sleep and nutrition and recovery, without the promise of any playing time at all… this was an opportunity to employ toughness every day, and to develop resilience throughout an entire season.

Was it tough? Without a doubt.

Tough…. More like agonizing; demoralizing, and oppressive. It threatened to break me.

But I could choose to let it break me, or I could persevere and fight.

I worked my butt off every day.

I invested my very being and my soul into the program.

But I was given no reward; no tangible accolade.

I stood on the sideline for many minutes. I stood on the outside of the white lines for longer than I wanted. I heard other players' names get called by Coach for their time to sub in, and I waited for my own to get called. Sometimes, my name was never called. There were some games in which I never got to step inside the white lines.

I had to hide my emotions during those games. After the games in which I didn't play, I remember going back to the locker room with the team. But instead of going out for food and relaxing as my teammates did, I would grab my running shoes and cleats and run to the practice fields. The back practice fields were peaceful and dark at night; they were completely unlit. I would open the huge rusted lockbox that contained the bagged up soccer balls. I would take out a bag, and carry it onto the field. The light of the moon helped me to see, but all I really needed to identify was the goal frame and the soccer balls at my feet. I strained my eyes to gauge my distance to the goal, and lined up the soccer balls. I whacked those soccer balls as hard as I could towards the net; hoping to kick out my pain, hurt, frustration, and anger. I fought so hard during game time to stay positive and encouraging towards my teammates who were able to play and battle during the game. Now I was free to release how I truly felt. No one was watching. No one could see my pain and emotions be released. The injustice of not stepping onto the game field just hours earlier could now be expressed. I had been positive for 90 minutes, despite how frustrated I was internally. I had smiled and hugged and celebrated with my teammates after a win which I had no * direct* part of. And I could not be selfish - the game was never about #7 getting onto the field; it was about MWS playing to a standard. It was about who we were as a team... and I valued that identity over my personal feelings. Over my hard work. Over my investment. So, I had to deny my personal feelings. I was a part of something larger than myself.

But my heart still hurt.

So, here I found myself. I struck so many soccer balls with bitter force, under the cover of darkness. No one could see me struggle. No one could watch me express my emotions. I struck ball after ball as I cried hot tears. I was hoping to let the tears wash away the pain that gripped my heart. Once my quad muscles were burning with fatigue from countless shots taken, I would possess the ball at my feet. I dribbled and performed cuts and turns over and over; right foot, left foot, back to the right again. I would train and spill tears on the back practice field, lit only by the stars and moon overhead. I would train until I had no exertion left. I concluded the "upset" sessions with a prayer. No matter how I felt in the moment, I was always thankful. I had the chance to play soccer, to be trained by a Coach and staff who cared about me as a person and as an athlete, to have the deepest of relationships, to be challenged....I had to remember that being at Messiah was NOT ABOUT ME. It was about so much more. And only when I was exhausted emotionally and mentally could I finally bring myself to my underlying condition of quiet gratitude.

After the snotty prayer, I would bag up the balls and put them back in the bin. I would untie my cleats and lace up my running shoes, and run back to the locker room.

Sorry Coach, I may have accidentally lost a ball or two during those late night sessions.

The practice field took the brunt of how tough it was to remain resilient to my purpose, and my integrity to play to a standard. I had to fight to remain steadfast in my purpose to play for the One who defined me, and to play for the team; both of which far greater than myself.

Resilience is hard. But it is a powerful character trait. As it is developed, it enables you to raise the expectations you have for yourself. It enables you to conquer a fear, to embrace struggle for a greater purpose. It is a tool that has power and influence; with no prerequisite of authority, of position, or status. Resilience is a choice, and it often is forged through difficulty. Its presence is known through behavior and carries wisdom and leadership for those who endeavor to practice it.

Choose wisely as to the necessity of toughness. As you embrace toughness, seek to grow your capacity to endure. The choice to be resilient may not be recognized by others. To some, your struggle may seem juvenile. During his own trials, Victor Frankl observed that "no man should judge unless he asks himself in absolute honesty whether in a similar situation he might not have done the same" (Frankl, 2006, p. 48).

Others' perceptions and judgement will never be satisfied. Chasing the approval or the stamp of recognition for your resilience from others is wasted effort. Embracing resilience through discipline is a personal choice, every single day. In your practice of resilience, you may even stir up feelings fear and discomfort in those around you. For as you embrace what is uncomfortable, those that are lingering in comfort may become jealous or fearful. They may resent you because you are causing them to see where they are choosing to take the easy route. Revealed prior, you can become motivated through the responses that others choose.

Want to know how successful you are being tough, resilient, and embracing perseverance? See how many people you "offend".

Seriously.

People often choose to be offended when they are fearful, jealous, or when their pride is threatened.

Your being resilient might upset some people; because you are able to do something that they haven't taken the responsibility to do.

Let them choose to be offended, as you choose to be empowered.

Not having a fan club as you embrace discomfort may be indicator of your ability to overcome, to lead, and to succeed.

Through wisdom, be tough.

Through habit, be resilient.

And don't let freezing toes stop you.

CHAPTER 6

GO RUCK

If you would ask me to secure a backpack that is larger than myself, load it up with heavy stuff, make me wear big clunky boots, tell me to go climb a mountain…and require me to break down and do 50 burpees every half mile, I might just ask if I am also supposed to wear a blindfold to incorporate an element of challenge. A venture like this sounds like a great time! Tell me I have a time cap, even better! I am a bit of a challenge seeker, a risk taker, and a *slight* adrenaline junkie.

I admit to being a little nuts, but I am who I am.

And I am ok with it.

I love to push limits of my mind and my body.

For example, I scaled the famed Manitou Incline with a 15kg sandbag, nonstop, in just over 50 minutes. The Manitou Incline near Colorado Springs climbs a little less than 1 mile, with about 2000ft of elevation gain. Nonstop, with a sandbag, baking hot June sunshine and a broken foot (which I didn't know about)…ingredients for a great workout and test of mental limits! There were a number of other climbers either on the trail or peeled off to the sides gasping for air. As I plodded by, they would look up and offer words of encouragement - and a few "whoa girl, you're crazy". I would respond with a smile, and an emphatic "Thank you! You got it too! Keep going!".

It was such a great challenge, and so much fun.

I can't wait to do it again, without a broken foot.

I ventured up the Manitou Incline with my sandbag, not knowing that my right foot at the time was quite injured.

Even if I had known at that time that it was broken, it still would not have stopped me.

Once I discovered that my foot was broken, I knew that I would need surgery, and that I would need a long recovery time to heal. So of course I had to maximize the time I had remaining to be active and to adventure!

I ran a Spartan Sprint Obstacle course race at the Fort Carson Army base near Colorado Springs, on the broken foot. The course was perfectly unpredictable, with flat sandy stretches, with rocks and boulders, scraggly sharp bushes, and cacti! This was my last competition before foot surgery, and simply being able to run hard just one more time before the surgery caused it to be abandoned fun! I don't think I stopped smiling during that race. My foot hurt like crazy, and each step caused shooting pain. But I was able to compete, and that overpowered the sensation of pain. I just love to race; and I was overjoyed with the chance to race hard one more time.

I was able strain towards the finish. I was able to use my body to run, to scale the obstacles, to carry the atlas rocks and perform burpees just one more time. For I knew that this intense of activity was soon to be impossible during the repair and recovery process for my foot. That Spartan race was one of the most fun of races. And I placed second among the Elite Women competitors. It was awesome!

My foot was very much quite upset with me; but my heart and soul were beaming. I just couldn't stop smiling. I maximized my opportunity to go hard.

I somehow got a bloody nose during one of the obstacles (maybe rolling across some rocks for the barbed wire crawl...?). There is a photo of me during the race, smiling ear to ear and revealing bloody teeth. "Cute" and "delicate" describe my image pretty well in that shot. Just kidding. My dirty body and bloody face caused me to look as if I got hit by a truck. I think the Spartan media guy may have been a little confused at my appearance, but I was as happy as a kid in a candy store. Maybe even happier.

Finally, a day before my foot surgery, I had to do one more adventure. I had 24 hours left of my summer; I had one full day to be outdoors, to be in the mountains, to be on my feet. So of course I had to maximize this chance.

I climbed above 14,000ft to reach Pikes Peak on a solo excursion, while still coping with that broken foot. I will explain details of this trek later. I mention this experience simply to share my orientation towards pushing limits of my body and my mind.

Nothing makes me happier than to take something that seems tough, to take something that I might fail at, to take something that is risky, and to give it my all. Does "giving it my all" always result in success? Absolutely not! But giving it my all, *and failing,* means that I can learn how to give it my all again and this time with a higher chance of success. And I might have more to give this next time around, as learning what did not cause me to succeed now allows me to have more to invest in my pursuit!

Something that I might fail at, an environment in which I am not comfortable, a scene in which I am completely a novice…. that is where I thrive.

It's easier to attack a risky physical situation in which success isn't guaranteed; a situation that has a tangible outcome. It is easier to risk when there is an external reward to be gained.

It's much more difficult attack an uncomfortable arena with people, responsibility, ownership, and expectations; risk that cannot be evaluated with a quantifiable result.

For example; given the choice, most of us would rather do pushups until our arms give out than have a crucial conversation with a family member.

The latter of situations is more difficult; for uncomfortable situations within social realms that include risk cause emotions to rise to the surface. And there is no promise or certainty of the outcome. Risk versus reward quantification becomes skewed, as sometimes we allow our own perceptions, fears, expectations, and assumptions to govern our ability to thrive within the uncomfortable environment of uncertainty.

But let's take this concept and apply it towards activity.

Loading up a heavy backpack while wearing military grade "accessories" and traveling on foot from one location to another is called *rucking*. "Ruck marching can be described as transporting gear from one location to another while wearing a backpack. This grueling task is frequently accomplished early in the morning when soldiers are operating on little sleep, or at the end of a training exercise" (Jenne, 2019, p. 42).

Rucking is utilized as a training tool in military settings based upon field task requirement, and is a combat-centric necessity. Learning and training to ruck is a process, as is learning how to perform a proper burpee. Form and technique matter to both activities. Both require practice to complete well, both are indicative of athletic capability, and both suck. Burpees are hard. Rucking is hard. Terrain and environmental conditions cause rucking to be even more difficult. I consider rucking from a physical perspective, as a training tool. But I also consider it as a mindset.

I was blessed with the opportunity to work as a strength and conditioning coach at Pitt. My title was technically "Research Assistant", but my Certified Strength and Conditioning Specialist Certification from the National Strength and Conditioning Association (NSCA) enabled me to functionally perform my role as a coach. The research I was invested in was directed towards strength and conditioning methods for soldiers and tactical operators. The goal was to compare training methods in order to optimize efficiency of time and effort of physical training.

The tactical population must be fully equipped for all components of physical development and performance, at all times. There is no off-season and there is no pre-season. These athletes must be ready to perform optimally all the time. This creates a host of obstacles for the strength coaches, nutritionists, physical therapists, and other professionals who are trusted to prepare the tactical operators. The multifaceted physical training protocols used to prepare soldiers for tactical situations need to be efficient and simple, yet somehow include all of the physical criteria necessary for performance.

General preparedness and movement habits need to be periodized into a program that also incorporates specific movements common to soldiers. In order to utilize task specificity, rucking (carrying heavy backpacks or sandbags) was included into the training programs that I helped to employ. As a coach on the project, I tested the protocols so that I was prepared to demonstrate and implement the training methods accurately. I discovered quite quickly that rucking is tough. Especially for my 5 foot tall frame… loading, balancing, and moving a backpack loaded with 75% of my bodyweight was quite a challenge! But practicing rucking allowed me the opportunity to experience what the research participants would be experiencing during training. A learning curve caused subsequent rucks to be much more manageable.

My first go-round of a rucking task included a paced march. I was loaded up with a 42kg military grade backpack, kevlar helmet, combat boots, and a plastic military grade rifle mold for the 50 minute march. After the paced march, I was to complete an additional 2km all-out effort. Total time to complete the task was the outcome variable. Halfway through the ruck march, my right began to feel tingly. Fifteen minutes later, I couldn't feel my right hand. By the end of the protocol, I could physically see my right arm and hand, but I could no longer feel them. I was experiencing rucksack palsy. The straps of the pack were very tight (and ill fitting for my child height) across the front of my shoulders and chest. The weight of the pack and the tightness of the secured straps cut off circulation and nerve innervation to my right arm. I powered through and finished the protocol - I wasn't going to stop! But when I finished the task, I dumped that pack as quickly as I possibly could!

Thankfully, feeling and sensation returned to my arm, and no medical attention was necessary. This experience was crucial for me, as now I was better equipped to understand and aid the participants soon to complete the training programs. The participants would also be novices at rucking, and my personal experience now could aid their success as they too would have to complete the ruck task.

My role and involvement with the military project at Pitt was a catalyst in my future pursuits as a conditioning coach. This project's purpose was to use various strength and conditioning methods to optimize the efficiency of the preparatory training programs for soldiers. My desire was to use my academic progress, my personality traits, and my orientation towards excellence to increase the effectiveness and the injury resilience of our soldiers.

My position towards excellence and towards the value of a team spurred on my intention to be useful for those who have dedicated their lives to preserve the freedoms that I take for granted. I want to serve those that serve this country. I aimed to use the character and leadership development that has shaped me to relate and invest into those with a similar mindset of excellence. How I used *who* I am to better those serving this country became a primary focus; it's how I knit a *mentality* of rucking with the *exercise* of rucking.

I understand the mentality of rucking as a psychological condition, but it depends on a psychological position. One can only begin to ruck mentally (condition), from a foundation of confidence, preparation, and resolve towards a mission (position). I will expound on this topic in Chapter 15, but position and condition are important terms to differentiate here. The mentality of rucking elicits a mindset of a destination that has yet to be reached. It eludes loading up a "backpack" of supplies needed along the way towards the destination. The goal requires having a plan, and preparing for the demands of attaining the goal. The mental "backpack" must be loaded with proper expectations and efficient habits. It must be loaded with practice and with readiness. The journey will include stumbling blocks and unanticipated setbacks along the way (a psychological rucksack palsy).

How well you have prepared your "backpack" will be crucial in how well you can move beyond these setbacks. Just as packing a raincoat to prepare for a storm may add a little more weight to an actual backpack, adding the extra "weight" to the mental backpack to increase resiliency against unforeseen obstacles is worth the time and the energy.

How does one add weight to a "backpack" of mental preparedness?

Practice mindset, practice to reign in your emotional responses, practice being a listener, practice being wrong (for it allows you the chance to learn how to be right, and this is the path of humility). Humility breeds leadership. Become comfortable with being uncomfortable, and evaluate honestly your abilities to deal with hardship. Problem solving, effective communication skills, prioritization, and discipline are things that you can practice to load up your backpack of preparation.

Rucking is a process; start from point A to get to point B. Set a goal, prepare, and ruck there.

Prepare thoughtfully. Be intentional. Have a plan. Be humble. Expect to fail.

I learned these values over time as a college athlete, engrained into the small choices made each day on and off the soccer field.

"Intentionality in everything, including the little things, makes the big things more possible" (Zigarelli, 2011, p. 66). Achieving the "big things"- the goal - will not be easy. If it were, then everyone would be achieving and striving and risking more; but rucking is hard. As you choose to "ruck" in your sphere of life, your goals, and your relationships, be assured that you cannot control the elements around you. Again, you can control how to prepare yourself, and you can only take ownership of you. To ruck, you must carry your own backpack at your own pace. You cannot control the environment around you.

It might be "muddy", or "cold", or "lonely"... and your preparation for the "elements" will depend on how much you truly risk, you truly care, you truly value discomfort for the prospect of victory and of success.

At its core, rucking requires hard work.
Preparation requires hard work.
There is no excuse for hard work.

"You have got to handle tough situations - any time that fear or pain or fatigue on your emotions could keep you from your potential. The psychological part of the game [of soccer] is an issue of inner excellence, of residency, of bringing your 'A game' regardless of circumstances. It's an issue of rejecting the pernicious self-talk that says you can't succeed; it's an issue of setting aside your feelings to do what is necessary and right" (Zigarelli, 2011, p. 155).

You alone control your response, your preparation, and your perceptions to that around you. To remain disciplined, to remain steadfast to your pursuit of excellence, and to remain immovable in your resolve is *100% and forever* under your personal control.

As you begin to ruck, you may come to find that rucking will cause you to become stronger, to become more resilient, and to be faced with increasing opportunities to take extreme ownership. Whatever your path or your goal, you can decide how to "ruck" towards the manifestation of success. "Everyone has his own specific vocation or mission in life to carry out a concrete assignment which demands fulfillment" (Frankl, 2006, p. 109).

"Doing things won't create success; doing the RIGHT things will" (Olson, 2011, p. 134). Do the right things to prepare.

Load up the pack.

Then, get after it. Secure that big backpack and helmet (because, safety).

Lock in. Focus.

Set yourself on a rock of immovability and resolve.

This is the staring point of becoming a leader, and of influence.

Go ruck.

CHAPTER 7

THE DAILY CRUTCH

There is no way to properly account for all the things that I have learned from dealing with foot surgery and the recovery process. In fact, simply describing the various avenues of learning could be a novel in and of itself. However, I will attempt to highlight some of the factors that have played the largest roles in my personal development.

My background as an athlete has humble roots as a 7 year old recreational soccer player, complete with an oversized jersey and "sweet spots" over the laces of my cleats. Other 1990's soccer kids know full well the value of sweet spots to performance. Sweet spots and rec specs were crucial for success. Recreational soccer was so much fun, and weekends were always booked with games and tournaments. Soccer was my main sport, but my competitive personality was still present in other athletic endeavors. I proudly sported baggy soccer jerseys throughout high school, but also donned the spandex of cross country and the notoriously long shorts of basketball. Non-competitively, I loved seasonal activities such as snowboarding and sledding and shoveling snow; swimming in lakes and tubing down rivers and hiking up mountains; raking leaves and digging in the dirt, harvesting dead trees and stacking logs to be stored for firewood, and taking on any landscaping projects around my house. My hedging ability is still sub par, but those garden shears made me feel like a worthy landscaper. These non-organized and non-competitive activities served to keep me healthy and strong in my elementary years, in high school, in college, and even after college. Of course, the athletic side of me was rarely downplayed, due to paint ball fights and super soaker battles. And any activity in which there was competition always reigned over chores (such as weeding the flower beds and gardens).

After college soccer, I played semi-professional soccer for several years. Semi-pro "in-season" occurred during the summer months, which coincided well with my schedule at the time. Grad school classes and work consumed all my time during the fall up until the spring. Soccer during the summer fit my time frame appropriately as spring classes concluded. I was still present at the NMRL to work on my thesis, but I had no allocated time for classes. Thus, my schedule allowed time for soccer.

Until grad school, I had played soccer my entire life. After college, I was not quite ready to allow the competition of organized team sports to become a thing of my past. However, semi-pro women's soccer is a niche scene. I realized that although I still loved the game, my athletic pursuits were going to have to change. Soccer was going to have to become something I "used to be good at". After my senior season at Messiah, I ran a trail ultramarathon, and placed first in my age group. I loved it. I grew into the trail running and endurance scene as I transitioned from college into grad school. But I had to somehow incorporate a high intensity aspect to ultramarathon trail running to make it more gritty. Soccer is a gritty sport, so my next athletic venture needed a degree of grit and dirt. I was physically strong, mentally tough, and understood the specific physiological and metabolic components that I needed to train. My capability to create multifaceted training programs allowed me to step into a new scene - obstacle course racing. These footraces incorporated endurance, power, and strength elements. All the things.

I found it.

I found the sport I could dive into, train for, and thrive at.

I found the sport that combined mental resilience, dirty and unpredictable trails, grit, and toughness. I immediately hopped into the elite circuit of the Spartan Obstacle Course races series, and have some top finishes at some iconic races under my belt. I completed a 27+ mile obstacle course race (called the Spartan UltraBeast), in the Rockies of Colorado at altitude. This course was strewn with over sixty obstacles, on the Breckenridge ski slopes; and I placed eighth among the female competitors. I won several short distance obstacle course races, and had some podium finishes at others. I love the struggle of the obstacle course scene, and I even love the penalty of 30 burpees for each failed obstacle.

That's right. Thirty full and complete burpees (jump, hands towards the sky, then down to a full pushup) is the price to pay if you fail or do not complete an obstacle. You must break down and complete all thirty burpees before you may continue to race. And each burpee must be done with proper form. It matters.

Trail running, unforgiving terrain, unpleasant environmental conditions, burpees, hanging from high contraptions, and a beating up my body are exciting elements of Spartan racing! Each element offers a physical capacity to be improved. Upper body strength and power is necessary. Lower body strength is crucial. The ability to run fast for a long time on rocky/muddy/ unforgiving trails and mountains separates the top competitors. All of these qualities can and need to be trained. If I am to have any expectation of a podium finish, I need to train all of the things. The challenge of training muscular strength and power simultaneously with VO2max and lactate threshold motivates me. I love to train. To prepare for race day and prepare optimal performance hypes me up.

    I trained for various distances of Spartan racing - from the short and fast races to the ultramarathon distances. Training for races is more than just a passionate pursuit or pastime. Training reflects some of my personality traits. Toughness, resiliency, love for the outdoors, and the challenge of pushing through difficulty and pain are traits of mine that are revealed through preparing for race day. How I express aspects of my personality, who I am, comes through the opportunity to race. To become a better runner, to become stronger and more powerful, to become more functional, to decrease my risk of injury are manifestations of consistency and hard work. Discipline, focus, hard work, and ownership are qualities that I can express through how I physically prepare. How I can become the very best athlete that I can be takes various forms of training modes.

    Training also offers me the chance to put into practice concepts that I have learned through my academic training in the field of sports medicine. My educational background allows me to apply cutting edge and effective science that replaces prior training practices. I am able to practice new scientific principles for my own athletic success. As I test them, I can be more equipped to utilize them for the athletes I coach.

However, the ability to train, to adventure, to carry sandbags up mountains, and scale new heights were all brought to a standstill.

I suffered an injury to my foot, during a two day Spartan race weekend. I did not realize the severity of the injury. I knew that something in my foot was injured, and that I should limit the pounding on my foot to allow healing. But I continued to train and prepare for upcoming events and races. My foot hurt, but I have a high pain threshold. The pain in my foot never reached a point that caused me to believe that something very seriously wrong. I maintained very high fitness levels, and embraced cycling and swimming. I avoided running and jumping, so I used other training methods to keep my fitness levels as high as possible. I was training for a Spartan race in Colorado, which I referred to previously. This Spartan race was about 10 weeks after the two day Spartan race in which my foot injury occurred. My increased time on the bike and in the pool mimicked triathlon style training. I always hated the pool, but with an injured foot, I knew that pool workouts were a valid training modality. Training in the pool also would have allowed my foot the rest it needed.

In this 10 week period between races, I embarked on new adventures in Colorado. It was during this time that I climbed the Manitou Incline with a 15kg sandbag nonstop. I was having a blast-doing as much as I could in the beautiful and rugged terrain around me. The mountains called to me. I answered the call without giving much value to a slightly uncomfortable foot. But that slightly uncomfortable foot just wouldn't heal.

Something was just too "off".

I decided to get some diagnostics on my foot, just two days before the Spartan race that I had been training for.

The diagnostics revealed that my foot was indeed injured. Imaging revealed that the navicular bone in my foot was broken. Not just broken, but in two separate and distinct pieces. Apparently, it had been broken since the two day race 10 weeks ago. To repair the foot, I would need surgery that included two screws, a tibia bone graft, and stem cell injection. I was looking at a 4 month recovery process. This entailed various stages from non-weight bearing, slowly progressing to a very gentle return to weight bearing. This meant that I would be unable to drive for (at minimum) 12 weeks. I wouldn't be able to get to work. I wouldn't be able to go anywhere. Once I had discovered the prognosis, I scheduled the surgery as quickly as possible. Putting it off would only push back my ability to work.

My surgery was set for two weeks after my imaging results. I had fourteen days to be a functional human. The fact was that my foot was broken. It needed some major repair that would put me down.

My foot couldn't really become more broken, as two separate pieces is about as broken as one can be.

And now I was *finally* aware and sure of what was "off" in my foot.

This discovery was actually freeing. Now I could adventure without having to "coddle" my foot. Though still in pain, I was pumped to know that I wasn't making the injury worse. The bone was broken, and I allowed myself to believe that I couldn't make it more broken.

I sought to maximize the ability to be on my feet, to be outdoors, to be able to move. I did as much adventuring as possible in those two weeks. I ran the Spartan race, finishing second among the elites. I ran with abandon, knowing that it would be last chance to run for about 4 months.

The day before surgery, I climbed my first 14er, Pikes Peak, on the solo excursion I mentioned previously. I loaded up a backpack at the crack of dawn. I taped up my foot (as if that would help anything) began the trek up the Manitou Incline. I began at the crack of dawn, and reached the top of the incline as the sun rose over the horizon of the front range. I continued the excursion on Barr Trail until I reached the summit of Pikes Peak. Then, I navigated back down, logging in a 21+ mile trek on a broken foot. My foot hurt. But I was happy. I maximized the hours I had left to be in the mountains and to hike.

Surgery loomed ahead. But it had to happen, in order for me to pursue a career and to continue to be an athlete. My Pikes Peak hike was the last hoorah of summer.

This entire time frame was part of a larger career transition. This transition caused me to leave Pittsburgh and move to Colorado. I had made the decision to move to Colorado from Pennsylvania after earning the National Strength and Conditioning (NSCA) Assistantship Award. This award allowed me the incredible opportunity to work with and serve the 10th Mountain Special Forces Group (10thSFG) at the U.S Army in Fort Carson, Colorado. This opportunity was one that I was selected for by means of a multistep application process.

I was one of only three other young professionals who were awarded a similar opportunity.

Each assistantship nominee was expected to work for and learn from an NSCA certified coach, under a stipend basis. We were permitted to select an NSCA coach who possessed the Registered Strength and Conditioning Coach (RSCC) distinction. These coaches serve the athletic community across a variety of sport disciplines and levels of athlete participation. Each assistant was expected to accumulate a specific number of hours and task requirements based upon their Coach of choice. The Assistantship programs are offered twice a year. One assistantship claims the fall, with a start date in August. The other seizes the spring, with a start date in January. My intended start date at Fort Carson was in August. However, my injury delayed the start date. My ability to work at Fort Carson would be extremely difficult during my surgery and recovery process. The NSCA and my Coach at 10thSFG were incredibly generous and gracious, allowing me to delay my start date until January. At that time, I would be nearly fully functional.

The next four months were all about recovery. My foot had to heal completely in order for my reason for moving to Colorado came to actuality.

Until this point, I was living with my aunt and uncle in a temporary living situation, two hours north of Fort Carson.

My plan before knowing that I needed surgery was to move closer to Fort Carson when my position began in August. But the implications of a delayed start indicated that I had to remain with my aunt and uncle. I was now putting them out; as we had previously understood that I was only to remain with them for a short time. Instead of 8-10 weeks, I was now burdening them with about 5 months of dwelling in their basement guest room. They generously allowed me to stay during my months of recovery. And they cared for my needs so very graciously.

As I went through surgery and began the recovery process, I began to realize how grounded I actually was. I was stuck in my aunt and uncle's neighborhood, unable to drive, unable to go into the mountains (which still called my heart and soul every day, especially in the fall as the leaves were turning colors), unable to get to social events of any kind (without bumming a ride from my neighbors), unable to work, and unable to run/walk/use hands. When crutching, both hands are occupied by the crutches.

No hands. One foot. Two very sore and calloused armpits. Time to be resilient. Time to figure it out. I had to learn how to adapt. I had to carry a backpack, sling bag, or purse of some kind at all times if I was to transport anything anywhere. Making a pot of coffee now took about 7 minutes. I had to navigate around the kitchen without spilling water all over the floor or spilling coffee grounds everywhere.

Everything that had been easy and effortless before surgery now took extra effort and thought.

The worst thing about my new lifestyle of limitation was that I was slow. I despise being slow and inefficient. Now being quite slow and inefficient was my reality. And it was very frustrating.

Allow me to briefly describe the hassle of taking a shower with a cast. Things that I now had to consider: balance issues, slippery tub surfaces, a water resistant sleeve, finding a way to shave, having to sit, reminding myself that in no way can I use my right foot for balance, and reminding myself that my right leg must not get wet...a simple shower was no longer simple.

My normal shower time of 10 minutes was impossible.

Now, a fast shower was about 45 minutes. And that doesn't include hairdryer time.

It was an ordeal to shower.

Let's just say deodorant, body spray, and dry shampoo were God sends.

I wore hats a lot.

These are just two examples of how displaced from normal I was.

Surgery and recovery shook up my normal; in fact, *"normal"* escaped my vocabulary entirely.

It no longer applied.

I was slow. I was inefficient. And I was limited.

I had to learn how to adjust.

To be unable to run, to adventure, to be unable take my trusty sandbag on excursions in the Rockies, to be unable to take my trekking poles to new heights, and to hang up my hydration pack for the summer made my heart hurt.

But surgery was necessary. It was essential in order for me to continue on my career path efficiently, and to continue to be a high performing athlete. I had been accustomed to training *hard* every day, to training with intent, and to moving as much as possible. The struggle now was having to accept being less mobile. I was accustomed to being on my feet all day. I was used to being awake at the crack of dawn, coaching athletes, training myself, and finding new adventures to embark on.

I rarely sat down.

I don't like sitting.

I was only able to write this novel due to the fact that in order for my foot to heal, I needed to sit more.

Colorado lifestyle had been treating me so well. My soul's craving for motion and for nature was satisfied every day. I was satisfied; yet hungry for more.

Now, I was confined to a house. I had to spend my time indoors. And the highest velocity of movement was based upon how quickly I could crutch the concrete sidewalks.

The pause that I was facing in life hit me right where we are all most vulnerable - pride and ego.

My ego had to take a big hit. My pride was attacked. My hard earned cardiovascular and metabolic capabilities were going to decrease. My endurance capacity was going to diminish. Those realities were inevitable. In order to move forward in life, it was necessary. As I came to terms with my limitations, I realized that although I was indeed limited, I could still do *many* things. I was well aware of all the things that I couldn't do. But focusing on what I couldn't do had no benefit. My need to move, paired with my athletic mindset, caused my focus to shift. In addition, I had to embrace the advice I would give any other athlete in my position.

Change your focus.

Focus on what you *can* do, compared to what you *cannot* do. The way an athlete views their recovery and ability to restore their ability to perform has a relationship to the rate of healing, to the restoration of functional capability, and to the development of resilience. Focus, viewpoint, and mindset during limitation directly indicates functionality of an athlete once they are fully healed.

I decided to focus on what I could do, not what I couldn't. My number one priority was healing; which meant that I could bear NO weight on my right leg. I had to forget my right let existed; it was no longer a valid appendage. However, I still had a core, a left leg, two arms, and a back that could not only be functional, but also could be trained. And I still had a beating and pumping heart that could be trained as well! I was creative, and found that seated battle ropes, single leg burpees, single leg pushups, and pull-ups were all effective exercises to help mitigate fitness losses.

Being limited physically could have been used as an excuse to deny the fact that there was so much that I could do. So, I began to investigate ways to improve and to challenge athletic capability.

I used my brain to become creative with how I challenged my body. I did a ton of core work.

So much core.

Core exercises were the most simple to accomplish, and require no equipment.

My six pack became an eight pack.

Being injured was the catalyst for core strength increases, and other functional increases that were of lesser importance when I was actively training for races.

Some physical elements deteriorated; others were emphasized.

My core was strong.

However, I don't recommend going through surgery just for the sake of abs.

Not worth it.

As I started to become comfortable forgetting that I had a right leg, I created my own workout "programs". I did single leg pushups, single leg burpees, upper body exercises balancing on one foot or in the seated position, pull-ups on swingsets (using the chains for grips, and allowing myself to plop down on the rubber seat after each set). I used small dumbbells and resistance bands and blood flow restriction training to maintain hip and glute strength, even on my injured side. Some of my exercise attempts were complete failures, but I continued to troubleshoot new methods to make function, movement, and exercise components of each day.

A firm believer in discipline and consistency, I was resolved to continue to pursue good habits. A good habit for all of us is daily exercise. Simply because I had the excuse not to exercise was the precise reason why I needed to remain focused and exercise. This was a concept of success that was engrained into my mentality due to MWS. "Do I give in? Do I fight through it? We talk about fighting through it - choosing to fight through it - all the time because you've got to do what's best for the team" (Zigarelli, 2011, p. 155). Coach Frey vocalized and emphasized the power of a "fight" mentality.

Discipline now was outside of the realm of a team, but I chose to fight as a matter of principle. I chose to fight in order to exude the highest influence. How could I encourage others to pursue healthy habits and deny comfort if I was not willing to fight through my own excuses and pursue healthy habits too? I had to lead through example. That's what successful leaders do. "Successful people do whatever it takes to get the job done, whether or not they feel like it. They understand that it is not any one single push on the flywheel, but the cumulative total of all their sequential, unfailingly consistent pushes that eventually creates movement of such astonishing momentum in their lives. Successful people form habits that feed their success, instead of habits that feed their failure" (Olson, 2011, p. 52).

My habits, in the pursuit of success and leadership, mattered now more than ever-when no one was looking. I woke up every day (almost) at 6am. I crutched up a hill to a park and where there was a swingset and playground. I crutched up that hill every morning, and did sets of single leg pushups and swingset chain pullups. After the exercises, I would snap picture of the sunrise, because the beauty of the sunrise reminded me about the deeper meaning of life all around me. I would say a prayer of gratitude, sometimes out loud and sometimes silently. Then I would crutch back down the hill.

Every morning I logged in at least a mile on my crutches. Those crutches needed the Strava app to log elevation gain and distance traveled during the 13 weeks of constant use. During my daily excursions up and down the hill, I would nod and smile at cars driving past. I actually looked forward to seeing the "regulars". I enjoyed seeing my neighbors on their morning walks, and of course I greeted all the dogs that I possibly could. I was the happiest smiliest crutch-er of the neighborhood.

I was in a club of my own.

Some of my neighbors thought I was crazy.

I get that a lot.

Nothing out the ordinary.

Getting outdoors and simply moving was a highlight of my day. More importantly, getting outside and crutching was the only way I could be social! Often, the only interactions I would have with fellow humans came from my daily crutch-walks around the neighborhood. Seeing people, interacting face to face, offering a smile or an emphatic "hello!" was mentally so uplifting!

The "daily crutch" was doing more for my health - my mind, body, and my soul - than I knew at the time. Remaining disciplined, consistent, and pursuing exercise were beneficial to my health simply because it's a general understanding that exercise is healthy. Upon diving into some research, I found that my "daily crutch" directly affected how I saw and valued myself, as it actually served to positively alter my brain function and behavior. And, crutching was exercise, which resulted in physiological benefits as well! "'Green exercise', consisting of activity in green places (in the presence of nature), is predicted to generate positive health outcomes, accrue ecological knowledge, foster social bonds, and influence behavioral choices" (Barton & Pretty, What is the best dose of nature and green exercise for improving mental health? A multi-study analysis., 2010).

Crutching outdoors afforded me the opportunity to "foster social bonds". Low and behold, my silly and simple "daily crutch" was impacting me in a greater way than I could have ever predicted.

Crutching around the neighborhood and doing chain pull-ups were not always easy decisions to make. In fact, there were some days that these decisions were just plain hard. And there were some days that I didn't want to. Some days, my hands hurt. Actually, most days my hands hurt. The chains were building callouses, but at the expense of some bloody fingernails. Some days, my hip flexors felt as though they were going to fall off. My right leg was tired of having to be raised up all the time when I was "standing". My left hip was pissed off, having to do all the leg work (puns) and load bearing, which was previously shared by the right hip. All days, my armpits screamed at me as chafing and callouses ravaged my skin.

Some days, I battled being positive.

But the choice was always mine.

And I knew that my actions to prove excellence for myself could be an influence to others. That was my motivation. I had to choose how much I valued being able to interact with people and to encourage them. By fighting to be a semi-capable human and embrace health, I had a leg to stand on (literally, just one) to encourage others that they too could embrace health, despite difficulty. Embracing health was as easy as stepping outside and going on a crutch-walk around the neighborhood. "Any exercise outdoors is better than none. Exercising outside is also a proven method to increase consistency to habitual exercise" (Ketler, 2016). Based upon current research, crutching outside was not only beneficial to my physical health, but was a proven method to increase my capability to achieve regular exercise patterns.

I could still maintain the discipline to get up early and exercise as a good habit - like making the bed and brushing your teeth. I could still choose to attempt new workouts, movements, modified training techniques, and alternative exercises that could benefit my ability to serve athletes in the future. I was going to have to be able to work with athletes who would have limitations in some way. My current position was one I could use to relate to athletes whom I would serve in the future. I was gaining a perspective on a personal level that could be useful. Athletes with limitations would be able to trust me, going through the physical and psychological frustrations that correlate to injury, pause of athletic endeavors, and loss of hard fought athletic capabilities.

Learning and integrating perspective changes and shifting priorities were crucial during my time of injury.

My priorities shifted from what I could physically "do" to what I could mentally "do".

Learn more.

Think outside the box.

See people.

Value the unseen meaning behind motivations and identity.

What I was learning over this time of limitation was that it wasn't necessarily the "accomplishment" of difficult things that kept me from becoming dispirited. My defense against discouragement was the mentality - the driving force - that sourced any "accomplishment". "Focusing on the actions (the what-to-do's and the how-to-do it's) is not enough, because it's the attitude behind the actions that keeps those actions in place, and this is key ingredient in what separates those who are successful and those who are not" (Olson, 2011, p. 27).

My attitude every day was my choice. My mentality sourced my attitude. My mentality was directly affected by my choice of identity. I am identified by Love, in the most fulfilling and empowering way. A foundation as this enabled me with the power to deny discouragement. Love towards others (and exercise outside apparently!) are powerful mechanisms towards mood, health, and positivity. The most generous of people around me at this time, pouring life and joy and encouragement into my being, helped to spur me on in ways I cannot even begin to quantify.

The expression of attitude is behavior.

Behavior is patterned actions.

If I chose a positive and a driven mentality, then my behavior would follow suit. That was my motivation. No one else, no matter how much encouragement that I received, could choose action for me. I had to take *action* and to light a spark personal of inspiration. The tools were all around me. There was nothing I lacked - there was no excuse not to embrace action and influence. I determined the value that I gave on the pursuit of influence. How I pursued influence was with a joyful attitude, as I desired to pour this joy into those around me.

This was extremely difficult.

I cannot say that it was easy in any way.

And I could not do it without relying on the ultimate source of strength and power.

My faith and trust in the Lord allowed me to step into each day with joy.

But it was still difficult.

The choice of an attitude of excellence and of influence is tough. It is hard to do things for a greater good when circumstances tease us to lose focus. The temptation to focus on comfort and deny the stretching process of adversity can overshadow, minimize, and displace the focus on attitude ownership.

Do not give in.

Work at it, practice it.

As the weather became colder and mornings became darker, my cozy bed was way more difficult to leave. The daily crutch, single leg pushups on concrete, and pull-ups on chains became a more difficult choice. Nothing was worse than gripping cold chains and attempting to force my 10 chilly fingers to cooperate, to grip those iron links, and to pull myself up over and over. But I simply couldn't allow myself to pull the comforter back over my shoulders and turn my alarm off. I had nothing to prove to anyone. But I had everything to prove to myself.

No one was ever watching. No one would have cared if I didn't actually get up. No one would really care if did one less pull-up or pushup than usual. No one would be really be affected at all. But that didn't matter. My motives did not reside in approval or recognition or acknowledgment of anyone.

Why did I crutch up the hill and why did I do pullups? Because I could. I was doggedly focused on what I could do. Single leg pushups and pull-ups were two things I could do. Walking was something I couldn't. Driving was something I couldn't. Walking was a reality I longed for, as was driving. But I could improve myself, despite limitation.

In fact, the physical and the psychological benefits of pull-ups are massively more beneficial than walking. Check this out. Pull-ups are one of the *most effective* exercises from a time and functional perspective, according to a recent article in the _Epoch Times_ (Milner, 2019).

From a physical perspective, pull-ups are super difficult, and they require time to increase proficiency and eventual success. Try doing them on a swing. It is quite humbling. I started my chain pull-up capability with simply holding on to the chains in an L-sit position. Just holding on for as long as I could was how I began. I would hold on for as long as possible. Then rest for thirty seconds. Then I would reach up, pull, and hold. I would do ten sets of holds every day. Then, I began to gain the strength to actually pull myself up, and lower myself down. I slowly got stronger. I became able to do more. And rest less. Eventually, I was able to do multiples of ten at a time. Towards the end of my most severely limited phase, I had practiced and trained enough so that I could perform 100 chain pull-ups in under seven minutes and thirty seconds. And I simply began with hanging onto chains. I began with a determination to hold onto those chains, and I began with a determination to hang on to discipline too.

Despite their difficulty, pull-ups are one of the easiest movements to train. "With access to a good bar [in my case, a swingset] and enough perseverance, anyone can grab the benefits" (Milner, 2019).

As I woke up and was challenged with the choice to crutch up to the swingset, I had to face the reality that there was no excuse to justify not practicing pull-ups. Other than personal discomfort of course; which simply is not valid.

A swing set, a pull-up.

Simple.

Personal discomfort has no place in the pursuit of excellence; even when the temptation to justify a caveat is present. Through discipline, with small and simple choices, one can experience success and freedom. Various stages of my life have echoed a key principle to success.

Keep it simple.

"Successful people do simple things that are easy to do. Because they are all also easy not to do, and while anyone could do them, most won't. Successful people do what unsuccessful people are unwilling to do" (Olson, 2011). To be disciplined takes various forms amidst the constantly evolving phases of life. But the principle of discipline is consistent with challenging yourself beyond your comfort zone. As I practiced pull-ups, the better I became at them. The repetitions - over time - caused my strength to increase.

Better grip strength, tougher and calloused hands, and a stronger mind resulted from practicing pull-ups. These gains are in line with previous research, linking physical capabilities of a pull-up to the invisible (and more influential) benefits of pull-ups. "The stronger our grip, the better hold we tend to have on life" (Milner, 2019).

My injury timeout was a hard diversion to my comfort zone. It was, quite frankly, a big ole pain in the butt. But the reality of the situation posed two options. I could choose to justify excuses and rationalize being "average" during the 4 month recovery. Conversely, I could choose to maximize the opportunity of discomfort. I had a unique chance to see how far I could stretch myself. I preferred the latter.

I was stretched indeed.

I wasn't actually stretched in a physical sense.

I am still about as flexible as a rock.

I need a yogi in my life.

But I digress.

There were some days in which disheartenment attempted to meddle into my attitude, threatening my choices of emotions. The days of incredibly limited social interaction were the most difficult. On those days, the value of intentionality became imperative. I had to step away from my own thoughts, by focusing my efforts on something greater than myself. The best antidote was to preoccupy my mind with gratitude.

Being grateful for humans, for life, for an ever present and loving God, and for social interaction had to become actualized. I would write a friend a note of encouragement; or I would go outside and crutch the sidewalks, or I would simply send a text of support to someone. Being grateful for a functional body meant that I could still go outside in the back yard, armed with resistance bands and massive 5lb dumbbells, to do a core workout in the sunshine. Being grateful for a voice meant that I could make a phone call, even if I really didn't feel like talking. Being grateful meant that I could sing praise and worship songs, even if my heart wasn't 100% bought in to uplifting tunes that day.

The power of speaking, and even of singing, can uplift the soul.

A preoccupation with gratitude lifted my spirits.

A shift in focus changed the game.

By acting from a position of gratitude, I could nullify the looming presence of the blues.

If you are thinking and feeling thoughts that you aren't a fan of, the solution is simple: have another thought.

And go outside.

Choose a preoccupation with gratitude.

Choose to focus on what you *can* do, and on what you *can* control.

Keep it simple. Be thankful.

"Spending time outside in nature also decreases obsessive and negative thoughts" (Ketler, 2016). It all revolves around your choices. No one else can choose your thoughts, your emotions, your behavior. Interactions with humans, ability to be in community with others, and gratitude are uncomplicated. Your habits are your choices. Your thoughts, attitudes, and behavior can cause your mind to shift.

Moments of discomfort are opportunities.

And maybe, just maybe, despite discomfort, the simplicity of habitual willingness to do the right simple things could propel you forward.

And maybe, just maybe, you'll increase your grip strength on life too.

CHAPTER 8

PHILOSOPHY, PHYSIOLOGY, PHOBIA.

What is your biggest fear? My biggest fear as a child was that Darth Maul from <u>Star Wars: The Phantom Menace</u> was hiding under my bed. Each time that I had to get out of bed in the middle of the night to go to the bathroom, I would jump out of bed as far as I could leap, so that Darth's outstretched hands were unable to reach my ankles. If I successfully evaded his reach when I hopped from the bed, my return to bed would require thoughtful tactics. I would approach my bed from afar, and with all the power I could generate, leap from the floor into the safety of my blankets. Sometimes I took a running start to make sure I could jump from a distance onto the bed to evade Darth's reach.

Darth Maul is a frightening character, but his countenance is no longer my greatest fear. My fears have morphed over the years. My biggest fear in my current phase of emerging adulthood is the fear of social isolation. The fear of being alone; no one to pour joy and life into, no one to influence…this scares me greatly.

My fear of limited social interaction became a reality during my time of injury and recovery. During this process, I was unable to drive, to work, and to get myself into a social environment. This period of limited function was about 3 months. During this time, my way out of the house was only through the generosity of my aunt and uncle, and my neighbors who offered to cart my sorry butt around if I needed to go somewhere. I was so richly blessed by them, for they literally made all the difference in my ability to maintain sanity. I was a new resident to Colorado, therefore my social circle was quite small. To see and interact with my neighbors were highlights of the day, and these interactions were the only defense I had against my greatest fear. I am to this day ever thankful for my neighbors and my aunt and uncle for their role in my life during that difficult phase. Without them, I do not know how I would have embraced resilience to pursue excellence amidst the physical and psychological adversity.

To aid in the healing process, and to mitigate the onset of psychological staleness, I was granted the chance to travel home to the countryside of Pennsylvania. I was refreshed by being around everything that was familiar; a scene I had been away from for years. My family and friends, the serenity of the country, and the values of simplicity were comforting in many ways. However, being out in the country, I was very isolated. There were some days when I hardly spoke a word to anyone at all; nor did I see many other humans to communicate with. Rural PA doesn't exactly have sidewalks to link farms to neighboring homes. I could have crutched on the main roads, but I think I would hinder the progress of the horse and buggies.

I also would have no way to explain to my surgical team if an injury occurred while crutch-racing the buggies.

I refrained from such ventures.

Instead, I still crutched a mile every day, but I did so by simply doing laps up and down my driveway.

Over and over.

My capability to exercise was unhindered. I was creative as I invented opportunities to incorporate fitness into each day. I found a large construction chain in my dad's workshop. I carried the 30lb chain down to the front yard, where I slung it over the wooden horizontal beam the love-seat style swingset. The chain draped over the beam, and it offered the same pull-up opportunities as did chain pull-ups in Colorado. The front yard also offered the most beautiful of landscapes to view while performing core workouts on the grass.

Driveway, swingset, and yard...my gym scene was complete.

Exercise form and technique were critiqued by my coaches... who were my super athletic dogs who looked on to my activities in the yard.

To distract myself while doing yard workouts, I watched the dogs wrestle and play. They were my entertainment and my company. They helped long minutes of core and isometric exercises go by just a little bit faster.

Exercise, nature, and comfort of home were helpful over the long recovery process. Still, the toughest days of recovery were those void of social interaction. This revelation caused me to question the effect of relationship and social wellbeing upon health and emotional dispositions.

Could there be a link between relationships and health? Is there a correlation between our biological function as cellular organisms and our social vigor?

I personally experienced alterations to my mental wellbeing due to social interaction. I am convinced of a bond among relationships, nature, exercise, and mood on physical health. The function of our minds and biology is affected by the our social and our natural environment. The limitations I experienced caused a decrease in my social interactions to a greater extent than it decreased my ability to exercise. It is widely known the value of exercise and its benefit to mood, energy, and self esteem. This knowledge caused me to be as driven as possible to continue to pursue exercise, simply to move. Pursuing physical health was difficult, but I found creative, effective, and simple ways to work out. Like using a swing for pull-ups. Like using the floor for single leg pushups. Like using a yard (or my bedroom floor if the grass was wet) for core workouts. Like using any flat (ish) surface for single leg burpees...creativity allowed exercise capability to be a reality. But creativity and swing sets could not mitigate the loss of social interaction. The decline of social encounters had a great impact on my ability to choose to focus on hope, joy, and purpose. The injury caused a revelation. I realized that being a human isn't necessarily defined by cells, by biology, or by mitochondrial function. "Being human always points, and is directed to something, to someone, other than oneself – be it a meaning to fulfill or another human being to encounter. The more one forgets himself - by giving himself to a cause to serve or another person to love- the more human he is and the more he actualizes himself" (Frankl, 2006, p. 111).

Meaning in life is defined by love for humans; as opposed to meaning defined by cellular function. This concept is supported by Dr. Len Saputo, M.D. "What we think and feel has profound effects on our biochemistry and physiology; an enormous, growing mass of research documents the ways in which our thoughts and feelings regulate the internal pharmacy of the body-through modulation of the secretin of hormones, endorphins, neurotransmitters, and growth factors, as well their effect on energy production, blood flow, and much more" (Saputo & Belitsos, 2009, p. 81-82).

"Mood and self esteem are known to be protective against long term health threats" (Barton & Pretty, What is the best dose of nature and green exercise for improving mental health? A multi-study analysis., 2010). It is clear that exercise is beneficial for the body and the mind.

But there must be more.

There must be an interaction between our social selves, and the thoughts that have have about ourselves, and the efficiency of our biological processes.

The direction of our focus creates an opportunity for physical performance advancements.

The focus on internal processing can have an effect on athletic performance. Research conducted on the effect of listening to music and running performance revealed that listening to motivational music and the attention that was directed to the music caused the athletes' brains to be unaware of the exercise intensity. This research indicated that there is an emotional response to exercise, through tracking the function of the prefrontal cortex, just by the attention given to listening to music. The ability of the athlete to direct their attention to the music, which resulted in an emotional response to internal stimuli, caused an effect on their performance. The external influences of the exercise intensity were down regulated due to a mechanism within the brain that shifted attention (Bigliassi, León-Domínguez, Buzzachera, Barreto-Silva, & Altimari, 2015).

We are capable of shifting our attention.
Both through choice and through physiology.
Prioritization directs our attention.

The research presented regarding both exercise in nature and regarding attentional shifting reveals a correlation between what we choose focus on and how we choose to respond to our external surroundings. Unaware of the current research that validates the link between psychology and biology, Frankl described that this relationship was crucial to human survival. "Those who know how close the connection is between the state of mind of a man – his courage and hope, or lack of them – and the state of immunity of his body will understand that the sudden loss of hope and courage can have a deadly effect.. when expectations do not happen… "(Frankl, 2006, p. 75).

Frankl mentions hope and courage, which are examples of attitudes. Hope and courage are always available choices, and they could be the antidote to physical decline. They may even serve as effective medicine, as an agent of healing. And yet, in the medically advanced world that we live in, we seek healing and restoration of our physical bodies through means other than attitude adjustment. "Our bodies have the innate ability to simultaneously manage amazing internal factors that keep us functioning and active every moment of our lives – that is, as long as we don't disturb them with destructive thoughts" (Saputo & Belitsos, 2009, p. 82). Destructive thoughts are sourced by our perceptions to stress and our emotional responses to external stimuli. "Stress and anxiety can be lowered through aerobic exercise, which also boosts self esteem and causes release of endorphins" (Ketler, 2016). Our thoughts and direction of attention affect our health. Although we have the capability to think ourselves towards health, it seems rare that we actually take ownership of this capability. How and what we think, concerning ourselves and what we believe, impacts our very life.

The thoughts we have, the attitudes we hold, and the identity we possess affect the function of our cells. "Mood is an integral component of daily life and strongly influences feelings of happiness, appreciating the moment, coping with stressful situations, and quality of life. Mood is linked with physical health and is known to affect the immune system and the onset of certain diseases" (Barton & Pretty, What is the best dose of nature and green exercise for improving mental health? A multi-study analysis., 2010, p. 3947–3955).

Mood is a reflection of emotional choice. Therefore, our choices of emotions play a role in our mental and our biological wellbeing. The health of our bodies, the function of our immune systems, and our psychological wellbeing need our *ownership of choice* in order to function optimally. We tend to search for the "magic pill" that will solve all the problems. Regardless of FDA approval, cost, or side effects, we tend to place much expectation on the "pill" and its promise of relief. We are inclined to pursue options of treatment that include the least exertion.

The more ailments it promises to resolve, the more costly the "pill" is likely to be, but the higher the amount of hope we place in it.

Search no more, I have found the "magic pill".

The "magic pill" is actually free!

The "magic pill" is ownership.

Despite the fact that we live in a society where toxins are omnipresent, the capability of our bodies to function and to heal may be affected to a greater extent by our mental processes. Our priorities and attention sourced from attitudes reflect our belief systems. Thus, our belief systems impact our physiology and function. Where and how we direct our attention therefore influences the ease of which we can embrace positivity. Mood and self awareness are components to daily life, and affect our levels of happiness.

"Exercise has a physiological effect on mood, as research has revealed temporarily enhanced mood states post exercise. Enhanced mood has a positive influence on quality of life including more social interaction, improved productivity, and better behavioral choices. Regular exercise contributes to sustained chronic changes in mood. Thus, both self-esteem and mood are regularly used to assess the outcomes of acute-exposures to nature-based interventions" (Barton & Pretty, What is the best dose of nature and green exercise for improving mental health? A multi-study analysis., 2010).

The choices we make can propel us towards our purpose; or to a meaning that we believe is a worthy investment. Can we defend our physical bodies from physical toxins through belief of our purpose? I believe that our choices of behavior towards our purpose can directly impact our immune system. "Good self esteem and mood could be assessed in conjunction with health markers, such as blood pressure, cholesterol, stress hormones (e.g. cortisol), and inflammatory markers"(Barton & Pretty, What is the best dose of nature and green exercise for improving mental health? A multi-study analysis., 2010).

Tom Beauchamp, author of *Principles of Biomedical Ethics* (2001) holds to the theory of maintaining wellness and vitality through prevention and a strong focus on natural defenses. "It can't be stated too often: The cornerstone of a reasonable system of true health care is healthy lifestyle. This includes eating a healthy diet, getting enough exercise and sleep, avoiding stress, maintain a healthy weight, avoiding toxic exposures, supporting detoxification – and perhaps most important of all, having a meaningful purpose in life" (Saputo & Belitsos, 2009, p. 73). The discipline to believe in a greater purpose, one that drives our efforts and mentality, may have the greatest influence over our physical being. Believing in a greater purpose will direct our lifestyle choices. Those choices are the "natural defenses and prevention" Beauchamp refers to in order to maintain wellness. The natural defenses are lifestyle choices that we are all well aware of. It's no secret that nutrition and exercise are incredibly important to vitality. "Those who are currently sedentary and/or mentally unwell could accrue health benefits if their undertake regular physical activity. Additionally, benefits of this type of exercise would be enhanced if the activity was performed outdoors" (Barton & Pretty, What is the best dose of nature and green exercise for improving mental health? A multi-study analysis., 2010).

Movement and proper nutrition aid the function of our cellular function and prevention of chronic disease, and chronic inflammation. The effects of movement are enhanced by being outdoors!

Regardless of lifestyle choices, remaining steadfast to an intangible purpose despite external circumstances could supersede nutrition, exercise, and lifestyle for achieving health.

Purpose, and love for people, reaches to the core of our ability to be human.

"The more one forgets himself -by giving himself to a cause to serve or another person to love- the more human he is and the more he actualizes himself" (Frankl, 2006, p. 111).

A meaning that proves love for humans could be the key to health.

There are of course, detriments and setbacks to physical wellbeing. Preventative measures of illness are not a guarantee against disease.

The lack of illness does not necessitate a state of health. Careful attention to mental and social health can be preventative against illness. What and how we think is linked to our orientation and investment towards our unique ability to influence. If we believe that we have purpose, we have the capability to hope and to have meaning. How we tend to our internal selves can be reflected in our countenance, the way in which we carry ourselves. "We can be happy and fulfilled mostly by who we are on the inside. The external circumstances that we encounter have little to do with the good life. Much of your happiness comes from who you choose to develop on the inside. The real you. The spiritual you" (Cloud, 2014).

Successful people and leaders understand that the messages they tell themselves and their internal dialogue is a powerful tool in their ability to influence. As a prior NCAA athlete, I understand the value of self-talk, of visualization, and of ownership regarding my internal dialogue. Visualization was a tool I utilized to direct my focus towards athletic performance and towards encouragement for teammates. In order to lead, to pursue excellence, and to cultivate a culture of ownership, internal development is important. "Self doubt can be more debilitating than the misgivings of others. We can escape others' comments, but we can't seem to escape our toxic self-talk. The doubts proliferate, one giving license to the next. Eventually, we choose to play it safe… that is not leadership. It's an unwillingness to take the necessary risks to get to something far better that we are hoping for" (Zigarelli, 2011, p. 226-227).

"Self doubt, guilt and shame; these choices cause us to feel that since we have not been able to achieve thus far, that there is something wrong with us or that we are bad in some way"(Cloud, 2014).

Developing the internal life allowed me to embrace the risks that were necessary to achieve character and athletic excellence. The more effort I invested into the development of the gifts, talents, and abilities that I have been blessed with, the more meaningful life became. I firmly believe, through personal experience, that developing the internal life results in "the good fruits of relationships, talents, growing finances, and much more. In order to have outside life that we desire, we must seek God and develop as people" (Cloud, 2014).

And I still have much development to do.

I always will.

My faith and trust in the Lord is a journey. It is a journey that requires no attainment of perfection. The journey allows grace when I make mistakes. It requires a willing heart from me - to love and to serve.

The love and hope that I am defined by is my foundation.

I am loved unconditionally, and unceasingly.

Placing my trust in this love is assurance of my purpose. I return all of who I am, my meaning, and my purpose towards God. He is the author and source of life and love.

Faith and spiritual life is important for all of us, from an individual basis. It is integral in our physical health, but is a uniquely personal experience. Cancer survivor Michele Goncalves explained that "faith in a higher person is deeply personal" (Goncalves, 2019). Her ability to cope and conquer cancer was affected by her own personal spiritual journey, as she explains in a recent article in the *Epoch Times* (2019).

As we each wrestle with our spiritual progress, we must appreciate its role as inescapable to who we are at the core. To function in optimal health, the elements of physical, psychological, social, and spiritual all must contribute. Len Saputo creativity expressed it in this way: "Healing is referred to as a return to universal wholeness. We are indeed single and whole human beings, and at the same time we are integral parts, fractals, of an infinite whole that we cannot fully comprehend. Any given part of our inner life or our exterior bodily existence can be analyzed separately from all other parts, but we remain one unified entity; our body is composed of trillions of cells that operate as one, and we also have an active interior life in which progress toward the oneness of advanced stages of adult maturity" (Saputo & Belitsos, 2009, p. 247-248).

You are worth developing your internal self.
Your meaning is one that only you possess.
Break through the fears and self doubt that threaten to hold you back from meaning, from success, from leadership.
Connect with humans.
Appreciate being human.
Exercise. Eat well.
Go outside.
Darth Maul isn't actually real.

CHAPTER 9

SIMPLE

 I cannot easily describe how much I love the smell of a campfire in the woods, and the sounds of cicadas singing their nightly songs. If you don't know what a cicada is, it's an insect that is native to the eastern side of the country. Also, if you don't know what a cicada is, I am truly sorry; the sound of these insects is soothing and rhythmic. Similar to a locust, a cicada emits sounds when its wings vibrate. At nighttime when the choruses of cicadas turn up, a beautiful hum is heard. The sounds of cicadas remind me of summer nights at home in eastern Pennsylvania.

 Cicadas were loudly vocal during summer nights; as cicadas only emerge from the ground in the summertime. Cicadas are among many components of summers in the country that I remember fondly. Summertime near woods and farmland meant sounds of nature, smells of the earth, and activities outdoors which are less common in more populated areas. Each summer, my family maximized outdoor fun by going on numerous camping trips.

 My family would pack up our 30 foot long camper, organize the truck bed with firewood, bikes, and other adventure gear, and be set for days of outdoorsing!

 This is a term that is completely valid, used as a noun and as a verb.

I use this word regularly, and it makes total sense. Even if it is not found in the dictionary.

My siblings and I helped prepare the camper and gather equipment needed for the excursions, and we got our jobs done with anticipation of the fun to come! But only now as an adult do I fully appreciate the incredible amount of work that went into these camping trips. Each summer we frequented certain familiar campgrounds with other families and friends.

The adventures, experiences in mountains and near beaches, the memories made (most of which involved troubleshooting unanticipated mishaps), the collaboration with campsite neighbors when unexpected weather or environmental situations arose, the gallons of bug repellent used, the constant ability to find new experiences in nature, and new terrain to be conquered… camping was more than just a vacation. It became a staple to each summer; it became an activity that permeated my being. Even in grad school, one of my most fond memories was camping in Canada with my roommates, Jordan and Alice. We seized a rare weekend of freedom between semesters to travel to Bruce Peninsula, a beautiful natural forested area. The dark gray ridged and rocky coastline contrasted the bright blue waters that crashed upon its base. We were far from the congested city scene of Pittsburgh, and it was a vacation I will never forget.

It was the most unpredictable; and we were vastly underprepared for the events that transpired.

Allow me to expound, as I'll describe a few unforgettable events that transpired.

Eating cold Campbell's chunky sausage gumbo soup with a spoon fashioned by aluminum foil - shared by the three of us - was a result of a heavy storm that obliterated our campfire dinner plans. Our tent almost washed away, and we probably would have been the same degree of soaked outside the tent compared to inside the tent.

Carrying Alice across a stony beach for a mile, Jordan and I found a new way to embrace fitness. Alice suffered a sprained ankle as the three of us were traversing across a rocky beach. The battle buddies never leave a man behind, so Jordan and I took turns piggy-backing Alice and her swollen ankle across the rugged beach back to the car.

Attempting to remedy Alice's sprained ankle with athletic tape that we purchased at the only local grocery store within miles of the campground was hilarious. Our efforts at being athletic trainers were laughably futile. Our taping ability needs some work. Alice was a good sport throughout the entire ordeal. She was a trooper!

Showering by means of jumping into the campground pool was a lame excuse for getting "clean" after days of being outdoors. But that was by far the most refreshing swim ever.

Exploring the coastline with my best friends and geeking out over the views was the best of experiences, and I do not think I can ever go back to Bruce Peninsula without Jordan and Alice.

Regardless of location, campfires are essential to camping (as long as Smoky the bear and the National Wildlife Service approve). Prime time for campfires is when darkness falls and temperatures drop. This also serves as the perfect opportunity for dinners cooked over the open flame. Campfires are the unsung hero of outdoorsing and friendship. I remember chatting and replaying the day's events, storytelling, guitar playing, singing, and playing games around the dancing light of a campfire. Campfires also provided heat for the best of meals.

Steak and potatoes and corn on the cob were prepared over the hot coals of the campfire. The flavors of the lightly charred foods over a cedar wood fire was by far so much more flavorful than an oven or grill. Preparation and cooking required patience. But campfire dinners are worth the wait. We would grab the food and assemble everything under the camper canopy, where picnic tables were staged for the spread. The food was rapidly consumed - campfire dinners were the most satisfying. Five star restaurants were pale in comparison - the scene, the friendship, and the food of a campfire cannot be bested by a price tag or yelp review. No matter how full we were, there was always room for mountain pies and s'mores after dinner. Toasted marshmallows smooshed between grahams and chocolate is an unspoken necessity of camping. Mountain pies take a super close second place to s'mores. A mountain pie is similar to a PB&J. Mountain pies are characterized by two pieces of bread separated by a beautifully thick layer cream cheese and pie filling or jam (raspberry was my personal favorite). The sandwich is stacked inside of an iron clamp. The clamp is placed in burning hot coals, allowing the contents to "bake". The pie is toasted in the coals and flames until the bread is a lightly crisped and the cream cheese melted into the pie filling. These pies were are as messy to consume as s'mores, which made them that much more fun to enjoy!

I look back on all the camping adventures, and reminisce on how uncomplicated it was to have so much fun.

It was simple.

There was rarely any hassle about event planning; about hotel reservations, about organizing activities, about rental cars and itineraries. We cared more about experiencing nature, the weather being our only real limiting factor. We cared about being together. We cared about embarking on adventures that were created simply by putting on hiking shoes. A camping trip was simple; but it yielded the most of rich of experiences, the most fond of memories, and the most numerous of learning experiences.

I fondly reminisce camping to share an underlying concept of life, of perspective, and of leadership style.

Simplicity.

Keep it simple.

Simplicity creates a necessity. In today's society, there has been a surge towards minimalism as a lifestyle. Minimalism is simple; one does not need more, although there is the option to possess more. If one is in a "simple" environment, there can be a desire or a focus on that which one does not have. A simple way of living can cause a creativity in how to perform daily tasks and how to function efficiently. Simple living does not necessarily mean limited living, but I believe that simple living poses more of a challenge for function, for accomplishment, and for achievement.

Practically, it's easier rid a lawn of leaves with a leaf blower than with a rake. However, a person gains exercise and physical benefit by using a rake. A rake is more simple than a leaf blower. And requires no gasoline or battery - just a pair of hands and hard work.

Simple.

A leafblower is easier. But it may not be best, based upon wind conditions, yard size, and even one's focus. If your focus is to clear your yard quickly, then a leaf blower is the preferred option. If your focus is to remove the leaves and exercise simultaneously, grab the rake. Both modalities will serve to rid the yard of leaves. Both have varying levels of efficiency based upon one's focus towards the task.

The simplicity of camping resulted in abundant and satisfying experiences. To make new relationships; to share laughs and stories around the campfire, to figure out the best trails to hike, to fix things that broke down, to avoid getting lost in the woods, to prepare adequately, to do something crazy (essential to each trip) for the sake a funny story later, to be prepared with several roles of duct tape and bungee straps...the list goes on of simple things that were constructs of camping. The necessity of relationships during camping trips made the vacation more than just a respite from life. Relationships caused camping to be fulfilling, satisfying, and special. Outdoorsing performed together in an environment where appearance, performance, and expectations were of no concern, was easy and liberating. It paved the way for freedom of the soul and spirit.

It was simple. Relationship. Nature.

Simple to acquire.

Even as a college athlete, relationships with my teammates made my athletic career so much more than the sport itself. Said best by one of my heroes of MWS, Erin Hench-Musau, "If we were a TV show, our relationships would be the main plot, and the games would be the sub plot, not the other way around" [Erin Hench] (Zigarelli, 2011, p. 127). Erin mentioned nothing about the training, the tactics, the fitness levels, the player roles, the success of the team, or even her own athletic capabilities. Nope, she honed in on relationships. You don't know who Erin is, and her incredible career at Messiah. She won't tell you either. She would much rather reveal stories and relationships about her MWS experience. Her humility reflects her character, and her legacy at Messiah. Since she won't tell you, allow me to brag a little for her.

Erin Hench has three National Championship rings (2008, 2009, 2011). She is a National Champion Runner Up (2007). She has the following accolades within the Mid-Atlantic Conference (MAC):

 2007, 2008, 2009, 2011 Conference Champion
 2007 Rookie of the Year, First Team
 2008 First Team
 2009 Player of the Year, First Team
 2011 First Team

She has the following awards from the United Soccer Coaches (USC):

 2008 All-Mid-Atlantic Region First Team
 2009 All-Mid-Atlantic Region First Team, All-American First Team, Player of the Year
 2011 All-Mid-Atlantic Region Second Team

Erin Hench is clearly a decorated athlete; and her accolades speak to her incredible athletic career. She was player of the year...TWICE. I had the privilege to look up to Erin during her fifth year season at Messiah in 2011. She suffered a torn ACL in 2010, which resulted in a red shirt season and gained her an extra season of NCAA eligibility. I cannot imagine her frustration dealing with her injury and rehabilitation. However, I am thankful for it. If Erin hadn't suffered that injury, I would never have had the chance to be influenced by her.

Why do I share Erin's accomplishments? Because she won't. A decorated athlete as Erin is likely to share their personal accomplishments. Erin won't. She emphasizes MWS, not herself; she emphasizes the God she played for and the relationships that defined her journey. Erin has every right to brag about her incredible career. Yet, her humility takes precedence in her character. Humility sets her orientation towards the meaning of excellence and towards her legacy at Messiah. Her legacy, her imprint on the culture of MWS, is saturated with servant leadership, humility, and love for the girls around her. Erin's legacy at Messiah is one that I hope I had upheld and promoted during my time as an MWS athlete.

Erin revealed that relationship means more than personal accomplishment.

She saw me, a meek little freshman.

She made conscious effort to connect with me.

Connection through relationship.

Pursuit of excellence through community and humble relationship building.

Believe it or not, the simple concept of pursuing relationship links MWS to camping.

Sport or vacation...both can increase a sense of fulfillment, or a sense of contentment. The fulfillment and the satisfaction isn't manifested solely by the activity. It is manifested through the relationships that are woven into the activity.

Relationships require no prerequisites (no fitness training and no truck bed loaded with firewood). They do require a little effort, but that is a simple choice to make or not to make.

How does one begin?

Connect with humans. Make a conscious effort.

See and value each other.

Simple.

Life is messy though. And can be a little complicated. There are risks, fears, problems, and circumstances that confound the idea of simple as a way of life, and as a style of leadership. Leaders who embrace a simple style have discovered that a simple and steady focus drives their efforts. Life around them may be messy. But leaders who have established themselves with a simple goal, and a strategy to get there are more likely to succeed. One must learn to peel back the layers of complications. This can reveal that the things that seem overwhelmingly complex actually have simple solutions.

And most of the time, our very own perceptions, choices and habits, attitudes, and priorities are the heart of how we view circumstances. Our views can muddy up our journey or path forward. We complicate our own direction. We can and always have the capability to keep it simple.

A busy and chaotic life driven by high expectations can still be lived simply. How? Through a firm and established belief system; uncompromising in the face of discomfort or perturbation. Attitudes direct our behaviors; and taking ownership of our attitudes determines our choices of perceptions. By establishing a pattern of beliefs, a system of emotional choice structure, we can embrace *simple*. Clear decisions made from a consistent system of principles guide actions.

Being grateful and joyful are principles that govern attitude. They must be repeated in order to become habits.

Construct a system of beliefs and priorities manifested by behavior, and thus you create a lifestyle of simple.
You'll have your template of consistency. You'll be equipped to face the inconsistency of life's circumstances.

No matter what circumstances you encounter, you can respond consistently through the habit of joy and gratitude.
Habitual responses of joy and gratitude are powerful influences on our ability to live simply, and to mediate stress of the unexpected. Responses to circumstances with gratitude has been shown to be beneficial to mental health. It's science! How we respond to stress in our minds is reflected through our bodies' function. By decreasing our own exposures (perceptions) to stress, we are increasing our cellular and biological function through the maintenance of circulating cortisol levels. Believe it or not, relationships have a direct correlation to our health too. "Joy of giving and graciously accepting love is supremely satisfying. After all, many of us have come to believe that it is love that heals at the deepest level" (Saputo & Belitsos, 2009, p. 205). Loving others and valuing relationships is important to health, and to our ability to influence each other. Being thankful changes our mindset and action orientation. By living in the simple captivation of gratitude and value for relationships, we lead. And our own human bodies can become revived.

Healing and leadership are simple.
They begin in the heart.
They flow to the mind.

They impact through action.

Relationships and life pose a great struggle between simple and complex. How we embrace simple - with how we lead, live, and take responsibility - is revealed through our inner beliefs. The internal self that we are developing. Typically, the things that we cannot control are the things that we allow to take hold of our thoughts and perceptions. Choose to be concerned with the things that you can actively affect. Keep it simple.

Determine a belief. Act in gratitude and joy.

See others; check your perceptions, and take ownership.

Go camping, and make some s'mores.

CHAPTER 10

HEALTHY ENOUGH

Can we ever be healthy enough?
No amount of disease prevention can guarantee life.
So does the pursuit of health even matter?

We all know, and most likely have personal experiences with what it feels like to in less than optimal health. We also know and have felt phases of life when we were in better health. There is a continuum of health, and life's phases cause our state of health to fluctuate along the scale. I am going to generalize and boldly assume that we rarely remain locked to a static position on this continuum. Here is the question that plagues our entire society, in terms of health and fitness.

Why does it appear as though we approach health as something that can be quantified? Specifically, why do we grade and value ourselves and our state of health by a scale and mirror, and celebrated with visible images?

images that may or may not have several layers of filters

Health is defined as "the general condition of the body or mind with references to soundness and vigor" (Dictionary.com, 2019).

Based upon this definition of health, I venture farther: Can health actually be seen? Can health, on an individual basis, be tangible? According to the definition, "soundness and vigor " are descriptions indicative of health, and these cannot be visibly seen.

You cannot capture an image of soundness.

You cannot weigh vigor or energy.

You cannot touch vitality.

Health is not and does not possess an image.

Health is not represented by miles run, by kilos lifted, by pull-up ability, by resting heart rate, by BMI, by weight, by IQ, by our ability to accomplish. Read that again.

All of the above mentioned *can be* quantified, or *can be* seen. Health may include these characteristics, absolutely. However, these characteristics ultimately *do not cause* or *define* health.

But, the question remains, why do we still insist on BELIEVING that image, that visible bodies, that quantifiable, statistical, or numerical values, define our health?

The answer is simple.

Identity.

It's a problem.

Who and how we identify ourselves shapes what we believe about health.

Belief.

Identity reflects who we BELIEVE that we are, and what we individually perceive health to mean.

What we believe about who we are, our identity, is revealed through our attitudes, and therefore actions, regarding health. Alluding to the common (yet misguided) belief that health is equivalent to body image, we align our effort to attain "health" driven by this perception. The manifestation of this perception is reflected through our incessant desire to attain the "perfect" body (what does that even mean); for the approval of ourselves, of others, and of the fulfillment of "health" by what we can see in the mirror.

We think that we will be satisfied once we attain the physique or the image that we so desperately chase.

Is that why Instagram has countless filters and ways to modify a picture in order to be flawless?

Is that why supplement companies thrive?

Is that why the development of weight loss pills and methods are intensely sought after?

As we scrape, claw, and strain to gain the validation of ourselves and the approval of others, we fail to see that people around us are doing the *exact same thing*. They are looking around too; trying to gain an identity through the eyes, the fluctuating perceptions, and the fleeting admiration of others. Our perceptions of others are variable, as their perceptions of us are just as variable. We approve of ourselves temporarily, but succumb to discouragement; and in those fluctuations we tend to perceive ourselves and others differently.

How we perceive others changes based upon how we feel about ourselves. And how others perceive us changes based upon how they feel about themselves.

It is an exhausting task, to attempt to pursue health using a gauge that is never stable, never standard, never constant. Our perceptions change due to the perceptions of others, which are outside our control. We often *assume* others' perceptions, which is quite dangerous.

With a pattern such as this, can a destination of health ever be attained?

Nope.

It cannot.

Because we can never determine, or control, what other people think.

We can never control how others think.

We attempt to assume it, and make the mistake of choosing our own stance based upon such assumptions.

Chasing a conceptual goal of multifaceted health through visible "requirements" or criteria is futile. Setting tangible criteria to reach an intangible goal is incompatible. It simply does not make sense. Described another way, you cannot fill a balloon with lead and expect it to float. A balloon can only float if filled with air. Any solid or liquid in the balloon hinders the balloon's ability to rise.

The concept of health can indicate the pursuit of happiness. Happiness is the "balloon". We tend to believe that being healthy results in being happy. But in order to attain the unseen expression (health) of this emotional state (happiness), one typically seeks to achieve something tangible (e.g career, family, status, image). We attempt to achieve happiness through quantifiable representations. In previous chapters, I eluded to the fact that happiness can be attained through a pursuit of internal development. By caring for the uniqueness of who we are (identity), and the individuality we possess, I believe we can readily achieve happiness by taking care of that which we cannot see. And thus, actually attain health.

We all are at a certain positions along the health continuum. A confounding factor to health is that not only does it fluctuate, but it is incredibly multifaceted. As referenced earlier, health involves bodily function, spiritual awareness, emotional and social concerns, and psychological function. The nature of health, complete with all of its components, can be expressed in more pronounced ways that others. Each component of health also has its own continuum. Our mental function and psychological faculties may be in a more optimal state compared to our cellular and metabolic performance.

A new running mileage, a new lift PR, a good lipid profile, a low resting heart rate, normal blood pressure, positive social environments, and a firm grasp on spiritual awareness *can* become tangible expressions of health along the continuum. "Foundational systems in the body can determine an influence on symptoms related to presence of a disturbance to optimal health. These foundational systems include: mitochondrial function, methylation, hormone balance, gut microbiome, detoxification capacity, HPA axis, and the gun-immune-brain axis to name a few" (Nikogosian, 2019). Foundational systems of the body indicative of health parameters do not involve a physical appearance.

Metabolism and biology, psychology, social and spiritual aspects of life are constantly in flux. So, if all of these variables are ever changing, how do we improve our health progressively in the most holistic way possible?

We can begin with eliminating the inefficient and fruitless ways we currently pursue health.

Holistic improvement of health refers to the minimal presence of artificial medicinal intervention.

At its very core, holistic improvement of health begins with ownership and responsibility. Ownership and responsibility especially of what we believe about health, and about ourselves.

What you believe about health, as a reflection of what you believe of your identity, will dictate your pursuit of health.

Don't miss this.

Dial in.

Take a second, and actually evaluate how and what you believe about health. What is your personal stance towards attainment of health? Why and how are you approaching it?

As an athlete, my view of health is biased towards performance. Variables such as lactate threshold, VO2Max, strength to mass ratios, and specific workout schemes are additional components of my health continuum. My view of health is shifted towards competition and performance. Such a viewpoint welcomes an examination of my unique identity - what and who I believe I am.

I am a hard worker. I am driven. I am a perfectionist; susceptible to my own overbearing expectations. I am a risk taker for the sake of experience. I am a standard pusher. I am disciplined. I am an encourager. I am whole. I am complete in who I am.

And I am free.

I compare myself to no one.

I chase and seek physical suffering in the pursuit of physiological adaptations and character development. If I continue to chase athletic excellence, does that automatically mean that I am chasing health? Nope. Does my image mean I can perform? Nope. Does being 5% body fat mean anything at all for ultramarathoning and spartaning? Yes, it means I am not ready for competition, and that my body does not possess the energy stores needed to perform.

For most, attaining a low body fat percentage is the "I made it!" of their health pursuits. They believe that being "shredded" means "health". This is because when they see themselves and when they think other people see them, that all the approval has been won. As one who is currently in what people think is the "I made it!" of a low body fat percentage and looking shredded, let me tell you this:

I. Am. Not. Healthy.

In fact, my nutritional state is poo.

Here is a breakdown of the consequences that coincide with the ever so coveted status of "shredded"/ "cut" / low body fat percentage:

Because of my low body fat percentage, yep, I look great.

Because of my low body fat percentage, my hormones are jacked up.

Because of my low body fat percentage, I have problems sleeping.

Because of my low body fat percentage, I am prone to injury.

Because of my low body fat percentage, my mood is all over the place.

Because of my low body fat percentage, I struggle mentally to attend social events where food and alcohol are involved.

Because of my low body fat percentage, I am looked upon differently by people. Some are envious. And some see clearly that I have a problem.

Because of my low body fat percentage, my health is not optimal.

Hunh, so maybe "cut" and "shredded" have some implications that Instagram users aren't aware of... maybe there is more going on here than"image".

Let's not forget that a body is a structure that will deteriorate. A soul is eternal.

And since we cannot see a soul, we resort to choosing to value a visible body instead. We value a structure, rather than the true essence of human life within our souls.

Can I do lots of super cool things (like chain pull-ups and some cool core exercises) that reflect a strength to mass ratio? YES! And do I work really hard to be able to do super cool things, and to be strong? YES! And have I worked super hard for my abs? YES! However, there is a threshold; there is a place in which performance and capability need to step back in the name of biological, social, and spiritual function.

My spiritual awareness and internal development right now are at a high point. I am functioning on the more optional portion of the health continuum in that respect.

My fitness and my physiological function, as I am beginning to shift back into functional strength and cardiovascular performance, are also on the more optional portion of the health continuum.

My relationship with nutrition needs work. I am on the far side of suboptimal on this portion of the health continuum.

So, is being a high performing athlete with low body fat percentage, high spiritual awareness, decent fitness capability indicative of health?

Partially- but not optimally. I struggle.

Again, I am failing in the area of nutrition. Thus, I am failing in health. I need to become less cut, less shredded, in order to become more healthy. Who can fix it? Me.

I have to go against the grain of culture, our culture of infatuation with image, to attain health.

This concept is sobering.

As a society, we would rather celebrate and appreciate an image rather than an internal condition of health.

I am the only one who can decide when and how I shift my attitude and my relationship towards nutrition, which will cause an action and behavior to follow.

Physical prowess is only one aspect of health. My mental, emotional, spiritual wellbeing require attention as well in order for me to truly pursue health.

What if I have limited social interaction?

What if I need prescription drugs in order fall asleep at night?

What if I have clinical anxiety or depression?

What if I have an incurable disease?

What if I have complicated organ function that disrupts my ability to function and to think?

There are, of course, a place for pharmaceuticals.

There are drugs available, as are other artificial interventions, that can and do aid in preserving life. There are manufactured and synthetic prescriptions which increase the opportunity of a disease free state. Drugs and pharmaceuticals definitely have their place. The biological implications of just a small pill and the cascade of chemistry that follows blows my mind.

However, it is the ultimate purpose of drugs use that causes the distinction between pursuit of health and ridding one of disease. One does not necessarily need drugs in order to achieve health if one is not in a diseased state. Further, a disease that can be treated effectively with drugs might also be effectively treated with holistic interventions. In this case, drugs can be used as the starting point towards a more optimal state of health in a progressive fashion. The goal should be to progressively (if possible, based upon the condition) eliminate the need of the drug as treatment. The disease becomes less of a disruption of health based upon a a treatment strategy shaped by lifestyle and by attitude. Thus, we can pursue optimization of various components of health while at the same time alleviating the impact of disease. In this way, we take responsibility for how we become more healthy, and how we decrease the presence of illness. We can take ownership of our health choices, rather than depending on a manufactured product whose role is to simply to alleviate the effects or the symptoms of the disease. If we increase as many components of health along the continuum as possible, there can be an exponential increase in function and expression of life.

For example, one who suffers from obesity may change their nutrition habits to help their metabolic profile and effectivity treat the disease. Changing their nutrition to aid the maintenance of the disease can also prove to boost energy levels, and to regulate hormone releases which can increase mood and self esteem. See? Even though nutrition- a simple aspect of lifestyle- can help treat the disease, it has impacts over other components of health as well!

Lifestyle and health and belief are interconnected. None act independently of the others.

My athletic nature of pursuing and attaining athletic feats might be admirable and might assist in physical health, but it has limited weight over my actual attainment of optimal health.

Who we are, our health, and our purpose in life goes far beyond a quantifiable athletic measure.

What I believe about me, in pursuit of athletic excellence and constant pursuit of improvement, flows into how I reach for health while reaching for athletic accomplishment. I work hard, I am disciplined, I am joyful, I encourage those around me, I love each chance to move my body, I risk comfort for the sake of something greater. The messages that I choose to tell myself, the messages that I choose to listen to, are the ones that drive the direction of my pursuit of health and athletic achievement.

What are the messages you believe about you?

What are the voices you choose to listen to?

How much attention and value are you giving to the assumptions about the perceptions of those around you?

Honing in on this can completely shake up and re-define how you approach health.

Even better, it can allow you the freedom to pursue health on your terms.

Take ownership over the things that are hard to face.

Take responsibility to care less about what people may or may not be thinking.

Why?

So that you can seek to optimize what "health" means for you. So that you can embrace a confidence in your identity reflected through mental, spiritual, social, and biological function. So that you can be free. So that you can prioritize your energy and time, and cease the exhaustive cycle of assumption based attitudes.

Fears. Anxieties. Doubts. We all have them. Analyze them, and diagnose your areas of improvement. You can overcome them through changes in your perspective. "A key component of leadership and success is to be honest about patterns and to expose them [your patterns of thought]; you must choose to be convinced that you dictate your patterns…" (Cloud, 2014).

The patterns of thought you choose possess power. Your human nature includes willpower, which, when paired with a freely operating mind, can courageously conquer the thought patterns that may be hindering your pursuit of true health. You are capable.

You have the power.
You are able to conquer the perceptions of image.
Unleash your inner champion.
Win your own identity.
Win heath.

CHAPTER 11

BALANCE = BULLPOOP

"That's NOT fair! " is a phrase I *vocalized* far less as a child than I *thought* it.

Mom and Dad really didn't care about what I thought was "fair", especially when it was presented in an argument among my siblings. If ever a comment about "fairness" did arise, my parents would neutralize the conversation simply: "life's not fair".

Conversation over.

A mature response as this from my parents was not going to suffice. Justice among my siblings was necessary, and my parents were of no help lending their authority in my favor. Therefore, my siblings and I learned that instead of vocalizing the lack of justice among us, we would creatively seek revenge.

Disputes among my siblings usually occurred because we played outside in ways that were competitive. We managed a host of competitive activities, as seasonal fun encouraged our imaginations. Every fall harvest season, the cornfields near my house were chopped down. The corn harvest in the fall had the purpose of feeding farm animals (chickens and cows mostly), and therefore occurred in the late summer months. The corn for animals was meant to be very stiff and firm, as opposed to the soft kernels that we enjoy at backyard barbecues in the summer, smothered in butter and salt. The fields that were previously dense with thousands of crackly brown corn stalks and heavily laden with firm corncobs were now reduced to bases of stalks and chewed up crunchy leaf shrapnel. These six inch stalks still implanted in the ground can be likened to a buzzcut at a barbershop. The evenly spaced gaps between the rows of stalks were cluttered with corn, leaves, and chunks of maroon cobs. To those familiar with harvest season near farmland, this is a familiar fall scene. To my siblings and I, this environment presented an opportunity. Much like using tree trunks, leaves, twigs, and rocks to make tree forts in the wooded areas around my house, the "buzzcut" cornfields offered similar building materials for forts. Stalks of corn with heavy dirt-laden root systems served as the bases and structure for our forts. My siblings and I would charge into the vast field seize our claim homesteads (within 15 yards of each other), and begin our fort construction. Yanking out the stalks of corn, thick with dirt cemented onto the roots, and stacking them upon one another, we constructed solid fortress foundations - as though building sandbag barriers. We attempted to create forts, shaped like shallow horseshoes, that were positioned advantageously based on the slope of the rolling terrain. Solid foundations and geographical tactics were indicative of who had the greatest advantages. As we laid the structure for our forts, we made the forts opaque by layering corn leaf shrapnel between the stalks. This offered "cushion" and depth to our u-shaped walls. The height of the walls never exceeded about 4 feet, but their integrity was designed with the intention of withstanding the onslaught of force. As soon as we felt confident in a "strong" fort, the real fun began. Any wrongs the we had committed against each other were about to be avenged. We armed our forts with corn chunks, stiff corn kernels chewed off from whole corn cobs that were left by the farmers' harvesting machines, and of course, the heaviest corn stalks. The stalks with the most dirt still attached to the root unit were the most destructive of artillery. The stalks proved excellent handles to fling the stalk towards the other forts. Launching heavy stalks and aggressively pitching handfuls of corn kernels towards the enemies was as intense as the final battle in <u>The Lord of the Rings: The Return of the King</u>.

My siblings were attacking my glorious and indestructible "white city". And I had to defend it without the help of Gandalf.

The corn cobs and the corn kernels were tossed with emphasis as distractions or to inflict pain on the protector of the other forts. There were kamikaze efforts to each other's forts, in order to steal any artillery (stalks, cobs, and kernels). The materials to repair the forts and to re-stock the weaponry took time and effort to gather. The radius around our forts grew more barren as we ravaged the land for supplies. If one could sneakily steal another's supplies, time and effort were maximized! But there was great danger involved in such endeavors. Kernels of corn flying at high velocities leave welts.

Those welts felt so satisfying to inflict; not so much to receive.

Imagine it; three kids with massive corn husk piles. Three kids scrambling around cornfields with armloads of leaves and roots. Three kids ducking behind the husk piles (uh, I mean, armed and fortified strongholds) and tossing corn and dirt at each other... for hours. There would sporadic "timeouts" in order make repairs to the fortresses, or grab a PB&J (necessary fuel). But soldiers have little time for comfort, and war is a taxing effort. "Timeouts" were few and far between.

Being indoors was boring, so back to flinging dirt we went.

Of the three of us, the victor of the corn crusades was typically my older brother.

Ugh.

A few years older than I, he knew the tactical advantage of positioning his fort on higher ground. He knew that the areas of the field that held more moisture, and thus he knew where to find the most dense of corn stalk and root systems. His foundation and weaponry were therefore the cream of the crop (puns), compared to my sister's and mine. My brother's foundation was solidly packed with "sticky" dirt, causing his structure to seem impossible to destroy. My older brother was also about a foot taller than me (as most people currently are), and his gazelle-like stride length caused his "raids" to my fort and my sister's fort to be stealthy, fast, and effective. My older brother was definitely the one to place to your money on, if these battles had any significance. They were certainly less than fair; but nevertheless, the fun we had and the corn kernel welts we inflicted on each other overrode the lack of fairness. There was an overwhelming lack of balance in our ability to construct, maintain, defend, and attack our fortresses.

"Fair" was far from reality.

But at the end of the day, the lack of balance actually caused experiences, fun, and learning opportunities I still appreciate.

The structures of our corn fortresses appeared to be similar, but the integrity of each fort varied greatly. Age, experience, and tactical position determined the strength of the foundation. The tallest, fullest, and most robust fort may have been constructed with the corn "fluff" and have little ability to withstand an incoming battle. What each fort looked like had little indication of truly how strong it was, or what artillery was hidden behind its walls.

The visual appearance of mounds of corn that we constructed can be likened to the bodies that each and every one of us possess. We have physical elements- the electrical and chemical capability of our cells- that make us human. Our physical elements are vastly different compared to the physical elements of the life of flora and fauna around us. The complexity of willpower, choice, and soul we possess beyond our phenotype separates us from nature.

We have souls. We have free will. We have identity, personal philosophy, and emotions. These are woven into our uniqueness as individuals. However, we all share biological similarities as physical beings, as members of the same species. We visually identify with each other based on what we see.

Which is why we should probably avoid attempting to converse with grizzly bears and sharks. We can clearly see that their species are different than ours.

We tend to identify ourselves, in our own personal way, by what we see in the mirror. We all want to look into the glass and approve of what we see. We look at our bodies and evaluate, based upon what we see, our value. We desire more than anything to be proud of what we see. We nitpick, we critique, we examine everything that we can see. We grade our own identity based upon the judgement we pass on ourselves.

Let's tackle a familiar theme from another angle.

Just making another strand of the web between medicine and identity.

I am focusing on this due to the fact that this theme poses the greatest threat to our life and society. It also poses the greatest platform to achieve a fulfilled life, purpose, and meaning.

We are a society saturated by comfort, perception, and instant gratification.

As advanced as we have become as a society, we are incredibly naive.

It's so silly - we grade who we are, the essence of being human and possessing a soul, based upon what we can see.

Does nature need mirrors?

Do cute little bunnies, majestic deer, powerful bears, fierce panthers, and flamboyant flamingos compare their tufts, antlers, brawn, claws, and wings with each other?

They don't care.

They have one goal: survive.

Our survival, dependent upon functional biology, is dependent upon our identity and our meaning.

Using a mirror to define ourselves degrades our power and potential to influence to that of a lemur. Or a sloth.

Lemurs are cool. Sloths are chill.

But being human is cooler.

I know I have mentioned these concepts repeatedly, but identity and perception ownership are the most powerful choices we have as humans. Identity, and therefore how we perceive, has great implications over success, happiness, influence, and leadership. These are intricately linked. We tend to grade ourselves based upon how we think others perceive us; by the standards that we believe that they have towards us. Yet, at the same moment, they are doing the exact same thing, comparing and criticizing themselves based upon standards that they perceive are valid, set by others, or by society.

Lemurs don't know, nor do they care, if their tail has one more stripe on it compared to another lemur.

Ask a vet; but I am pretty confident in this claim.

Our structure of society has caused many of us to wade in a bog of bullpoop. Doesn't that sound lovely? You are drudging around in a smelly thick mire of messy priorities based upon fleeting perceptions and assumption. We are all in it, some knee deep, others chest high, others nearly suffocating.

We want instant approval from ourselves and from others.

We shape our identities based upon expectations and perceptions of others that may or may not exist.

We fumble our priorities in the attempt to appear put together and in control despite our inner insecurities.

We lack foundational stability of our internal selves, and therefore exhaust ourselves in our quest of identity.

Operating from a place of inconsistency based upon perceptions opens the door for fears, anxieties, and insecurities to have undue power in our decision making.

In the pursuit of positive lifestyle choices, healthy relationships, and a "comfortable" life, there seems to be a dependence upon achieving the approval of others to justify, to validate, to determine how we grade ourselves.

Let's stop the cycle of madness, please?

Perceive differently.

You alone control your perceptions.

Your perception of you begins with how you see yourself: your innate gifts, personality traits, strengths, and weaknesses. From here, you can begin to frame who you are. From here, you can begin to shape how you see yourself, and begin to operate from a place of confidence and consistency despite circumstances and expectations (fleeting, ever-changing, and dynamic) from yourself or others.

I challenge you to this:

Cease giving value to what you think that others may be thinking about you.

Actions based from assumptions about others' perceptions destructive.

Stop comparing.

Comparing steals joy, life, energy, and freedom.

Pursue being the best version of yourself, because you are the only you. And you, operating from a place of firm and abashed identity allows you the opportunity to lead. From an identity set steadfastly towards loving and serving others around you, you allow influence to flow! You will emit an essence that people are drawn to. Your meaning will surge from your very being. From a mindset of internal growth can influence and excellence gain momentum.

Life will always have "what-ifs". Life will never be predictable. Life will never be balanced. The future will never be certain. We justify succumbing to anxiety due to the rate of flux and high unpredictability in life. Why? Because we search for confidence in that which is not concrete. We yearn for identity in things that are not up to us; and we exhaust our precious time and effort into working towards security. We seek instant gratification, especially if we feel uncomfortable. We cripple ourselves in the attempt to stand tall. We have embraced a false confidence; because we choose to find affirmation on a surface as shifty as sand.

We bankrupt our resources of time and energy and innovation in the desperate and pointless attempt to build guaranteed security. Chasing security is as valid a mission as catching the wind. Choose to chase that which you can control - your identity. Only you can decide how you define yourself.

It is all a choice.

Take control of your own perceptions and your emotions.

Your emotions and your responses are always in your control.

What you have chosen to prioritize, to value, and to sacrifice in order to pursue identity, security, and happiness is always up to you.

The investment of your time and energy directly relates to the rate of gain towards success.

The condition of your soul indicates your position of potential influence. This takes daily attention and care. "Position your daily actions so time is working for you instead of against you. Because time will either promote you or expose you" (Olson, 2011, p. 46).

To cease hunting for the fleeting sense of security means to seize ownership.

Ownership is accomplished internally, but expressed by virtue of action.

Ownership stems from identity, which drives attitude; and therefore actualizes beliefs.

What you believe about you determines the course of your actions. It plays an essential role in how you build your life, pursue excellence, and seek meaning. Your personal philosophy drives your perceptions. "Your philosophy is the lens of your life" (Olson, 2011).

What you believe and the resulting thought patterns will direct the how and the why of your life. "There are two types of attitudes: entitled and value driven. Your philosophy is what you know, how you hold to what you know, and how it affects what you do" (Olson, 2011, p. 28).

You can never control the future. You can never control anyone's behavior. You are powerless to control anything other than your attitudes and beliefs.

Your powerlessness is actually freeing. All the time and effort directed towards assurance can be realigned and concentrated to propel you forward. No more wasted precious resources. Choose to take ownership of prioritization.

Your emotions are a choice. Your perceptions are a choice. Your beliefs about you are choices. The voices you listen to only have power you assign. No one can decide these things for you. Circumstances do not dictate these choices. It's easy to place blame, to justify, to gain comfort in placing responsibility on other people or on adversity or onto a situation. "The predominant state of mind displayed by those people on the failure curve is blame. The predominant state of mind displayed by those people on the success curve is responsibility" (Olson, 2011, p. 100).

Be responsible.

Do not allow circumstances to derail your mindset.

Seeking personal comfort and easing our lack of assurance deters the development of identity and character. Confidence and consistency are lost; influence is hardly possible. When we choose to submit to anxiety and fear, we give in. That is the moment we have chosen to give up ownership.

Taking ownership of attitude is not easy. Developing a solid foundational identity based on the unchangeable elements of who we are as individuals, as eternal souls, is hard work. It requires little choices. It requires focus. It requires resolve. It requires attitude. It requires action. No one really may acknowledge the actions, or see the effort that you are investing. Personal growth is not seen, that is why it matters so much. But then again, if you are doing it to be acknowledged by others, then your efforts are ill sourced and will not advance your goal. This is a reflection of an element of success called integrity. Integrity ties artfully into excellence. "It is not a conditional word. It is what you do when no one is watching. It is also doing the thing you said you were going to do long after the mood you said it in has left you" (Olson, 2011, pg. 90-91). Integrity is who you decide to be when no is there to pat you on the back. Integrity is an element of success that is rarely rewarded externally. Do not expect reward; simply embrace integrity due to its priceless internal value. Integrity is seldom seen. But those who practice and value integrity are the ones who lead. They are the ones who achieve success without focusing primarily on the attainment of success.

Evaluate who you are. Take up your identity, and move forward with integrity. Remove "balance" from your vocabulary.

Life is and never will be fair.

Be consistent to you.

You are the only you, thus, you alone can be the best you that you can possibly be.

What are you waiting for?

Prioritize and execute (Willink & Babin, 2015).

And choose the high ground in the cornfield.

CHAPTER 12

EMBRACE THE SUCK

Off season for most NCAA athletes indicates a period of time in which they (typically) relax. After a taxing in-season period, the off season allows sore and tired bodies to recover. The off-season welcomes a time for athletes to work on individual skills. The off-season for an athlete may appear as a period of rest.

I have no idea what a traditional understanding of "rest" means.

At Messiah, the off-season was the most fitness intense time of year. It was prime time for the development of team chemistry, as the younger classes now stepped into mature roles. The off season schedule forged the team dynamic, fitness, and culture for the competitive season months and months away.

Off-season training was hard. It included Challenge Days, plyometric and speed sessions, lifting, technical sets in the gym, and treadmill/road/ track workouts. Challenge Days were special days- they included a voluntary treadmill workout. Although completely optional, these workouts were expected from every teammate to be accomplished. We encouraged each other to do them, as though the workout was mandatory. The treadmill workout was to be done until failure; as many reps as possible, or for as long as possible.

We completed Challenge Days surrounded by one other. Teammates ran on treadmills beside me, and others would surround the treadmills and shout words of encouragement. The workout was to be "scored" on an individual basis. You were expected to run your best, and aided by the support of your teammates around you cheering you on, push your mind and your body farther than you thought possible.

Each Challenge Day posed a different workout, but each one was designed to be an all out effort. It was meant to challenge physical fitness, and to simultaneously haunt the mind. Why? To develop a mentality; a mentality essential to the MWS culture.

Don't. Give. In.

"You go as long as you can. Some girls figure out pretty quickly, sheepishly admitting: 'Coach, I'm not mentally tough.' 'I know,' he responds gently but with a chuckle. 'That's why we are doing this' " (Zigarelli, 2011, p. 159). The author of *The Messiah Method* witnessed these days of suffering, he was able to discover firsthand our reason "why". Our "why" was to cultivate mental toughness; to encourage us to choose to resist giving in to physical exhaustion, and to fight just a little bit longer for the girls running beside you.

Mental toughness is integral to the culture of MWS, and Challenge Days were a modality utilized to train it. Mental toughness had to be practiced. "We separate act from feel...do what you are supposed to do regardless of what you want to do" (Zigarelli, 2011, p. 157).

Mental toughness to stay on the treadmill; to remain positive despite having not the "best" run that day; to encourage teammates despite personal frustration; to run just one minute longer because teammates are worth one more minute of my lungs and legs burning for oxygen.... could only be real if I made that choice. I had to choose to deny comfort - to deny the "easy" choices.

Each and every Challenge Day, I had these choices to make. My choices before I even stepped foot onto the treadmill determined the maturation of mental toughness. To encourage my teammates when I really didn't feel like it, to cheer my heart out despite my feelings, and to genuinely desire my teammates to better my own performance was foundational to Challenge Days as the visible display of mental toughness.

It was difficult.

The workouts were brutal enough without the aspect of character development tossed in.

Challenge days were gnarly.

Choosing to push myself beyond my comfort zone regardless of my feelings or emotions was a challenge that burning legs and lungs couldn't match.

This was meant to cultivate team chemistry, through individual selfless choices. "That is what motivates people to maximum effort. Chemistry inspires. Mental toughness is your ability to focus on what you can control. If you start focusing on things that you cannot control, you're just as soft because you can't handle your world around you, so you start lashing out at things that take away the focus" (Zigarelli, 2011, p. 117; 122; 155).

Challenge Day workouts were oppressive They weighed heavily on the heart. They were so tough. They caused much anxiety. Even more frustrating, the treadmills we completed Challenge Days on faced a beautifully bland beige block wall. The treadmills were, well, let's describe them as "not new". The indoor arena where the treadmills were positioned barely had any air flow circulating. The air was smelly and dense. Conditions were less than optimal; which provided another stimulus to build mental toughness.

The day before a Challenge, my teammates and I would all talk about when we were going to "hit it" the next day. Who were going to be running buddies, who was going to be in the area to cheer on the runners inbetween classes, and who needed to visit the athletic trainers before their run were some of the logistics that preceded Challenge Days. We would hydrate and prepare nutritionally with *meticulous* care and detail. We were a bit superstitious about our Challenge Day prep. We would be sure to get to bed on time. Some of us would toss in some extra stretching and mobility work, to be as fully ready as possible to push our bodies and lungs to the breaking point the following day. The majority of us even had our "lucky" running socks, shorts, sports bra, tank top or cutoff, and pre-wrap. All the pieces that we could control for a "successful" Challenge Day were tended to with the utmost attention.

As anxiety producing as Challenge Days were, I loved them. It was a chance to see 1) how fit I was 2) how mentally strong I was, and 3) how much encouragement and camaraderie mattered as each team changed personnel from season to season. I will always remember Challenge Days with a sense of both pride and dread. The personal accomplishment of pushing my body to its limit; yet the dread of Challenge Day carnage included pain - physical and mental. An alumni of the Messiah Men's Soccer team (a program that also performed Challenge Days), described Challenge Days in this way. "We run. Learning to think about something else besides the pain, experiencing for ourselves the distinction between act and feel. There were guys who didn't think that they had a chance to make it but did it because of the encouragement. If they had done it by themselves, they would have hopped off. The last thing you want is to let your teammates down. Doing it when it doesn't matter carries over to the times when it does" [Nick Thompson] (Zigarelli, 2011, p. 160). The Challenge Day tradition from year to year allowed players the chance to grow. Fitness , necessary for soccer, was the medium to train mental toughness, necessary for Messiah Soccer. My accomplishment of Challenge Days instilled in me mental toughness.

Mental toughness means so much more for character development than running for fitness improvement.

Running for seemingly an eternity and gasping for air had to become less important than selling out for my teammates.

At the time, I had little understanding its implications over leadership and success. But mental toughness lights the way to character development. Mental toughness is crucial in order to grow, to overcome, to succeed, and to influence.

Challenge Days, and thus the very culture of MWS, ignited the spark of my character development. The struggles of Challenge Days offered the pathway towards the ultimate goal of the program - culture, consistency, value of team over individual, development of Christian character, and actualization of playing to a standard.

Just like Challenge Days, there are trials before us, and each one of us is plodding through it. Some of us are in a struggle, in a state of adversity, in a catastrophic situation. No matter what we are are facing, we can be assured that every single person that we encounter is also facing a difficulty. We have no place to judge each others' struggles, for each person has to bear their own cross in their own way. We are faced with the individual assessment of how much energy to invest climbing our mountains.

How we respond to our unique situation matters; and we all can respond with varying levels of resilience, tenacity, and grit. Viktor Frankl described it in this way "Suffering in and of itself is meaningless; we give our suffering meaning by the way in which we respond to it" (Frankl, 2006).

The struggles that we go through can serve as growth opportunities on a very personal and individual level. Yet, as we respond to our struggle, we influence those around us. Since we all share a common position of struggle in some way, we influence each other through the essence of relationship as we struggle. How we influence each other while we sift through our adversities is meaningful. Most of us seek respite from tension - comfort from the adversity, or the quickest or easiest way around the adversity. Choosing an "easy" path through adversity is always an option. But there is much to be gained through adversity. Yet the opportunity to learn, to grow, to practice being a leader requires a mindset that embraces the difficulty with a greater perspective of seeing beauty and value within the struggle and through the hardship.

When we are faced with adversity, we become uncomfortable. Discomfort causes us to question ourselves, and the resulting self doubt is the catalyst to action. Self doubt is a belief, as is self confidence. Both propel one to action. The action that we choose can spur us forward, or can maintain our passive current state. Or it can be a subtle expression of our own pride; often we are hurt by not being able to control our "world". Jocko Willink describes pride expressed through the ego. "Ego clouds and disrupts everything: the planning process, the ability to take good advice, and the ability to accept constructive criticism. It can stifle someone else's sense of self-preservation. Often, the most difficult ego to deal with is your own"(Willink & Babin, 2015).

We must check our own ego, and evaluate the realistic nature of our situation. Then we must take ownership of our response and choice of emotions, and determine a path forward that is founded upon hope. The result is an ability to rise up from the place of discomfort. Sacrifice is necessary in the pursuit of a goal, and typically that sacrifice involves discomfort, and a sense of uncertainty. "Whatever the dream, whatever the goal, there is a price to pay, and that means giving up something" (Olson, 2011, p. 161).

Your dream - to lead, to be successful - is dependent upon your willingness to "embrace the suck" of some unavoidable discomfort along way.

The ability to take ownership of one's emotions and make progressive steps forward is an indication of one's potential to lead. "Those that can forgo short term comfort due to a value in a longer term benefit increase their capacity for leadership and for character building" (Willink & Babin, 2015).

This concept comes more alive through components described by Dr. Henry Cloud. Characteristics of successful people include their ability to do the difficult things, in the midst of adversity. "These successful people have come to understand that discipline precedes strength, as investment occurs before a return". Even further, it is important to adopt the concept of "embrace the suck". I like to use this phrase, as it admits a feeling of discomfort, yet a determination to accept and to fight through the discomfort. In practical terms, there is value behind taking on something that needs to be done regardless of the high probability of pain or discomfort involved in that action. "The discipline to choose to face a season of pain, disruption, discomfort, effort, or something that hurts a bit is what people who are successful embrace with an expectation of a longer time of relief through that moment of pain" (Cloud, 2014).

In the society we live in today, the trend is to seek comfort as soon as something arises that instigates anxiety. The catalyst that causes us to feel out of control only holds power once we scramble haphazardly to attain comfort. We want to feel on top again. We want supremacy of control. Circumstances are powerless unless we decide to give them dominion due our emotional response. This can indicate weakness of character.

There is a link between our thoughts and our physical health, as discussed previously.

Surprised?

The intensity to which we allow uncertainty to govern our attitudes, emotions, and therefore, actions, has implications over our biological function. "The root cause of many mental health diagnoses, such as depression and anxiety, can be found outside the brain and successfully treated" (Nikogosian, 2019).

The discomfort and the adversities that we face, and our response to those adversities, is reflected not just in our personal lives, but in our healthcare system as well. Len Saputo, MD, alludes to the reality that "We are all mere humans whose natural tendency is to focus on any glimmer of hope for quickly ridding ourselves of our pain and our symptoms, without much effort on our part" (Saputo & Belitsos, 2009).

We attempt to fix lack of health with tactics that require minimal changes to our comfort. We desire balance. We seek comfort. We desperately run after instant gratification.

But many people don't even like the word "run".

It's too "uncomfortable".

We run - sprint - towards healing and health without actually wanting to put forth the effort of running.

Heaven forbid we exert a little effort, or sweat a little.

Curious.

We fail to investigate and to be responsible for things in our own lives that we have the power to change to increase our health.

We prefer to value a possible solution that flows seamlessly with our comfort, regardless of a holistic perspective towards the pursuit of optimal health. We prefer to bankrupt our resources for a quick and effortless "fix" or "healing". We spin our wheels in this vicious cycle, instead of valuing internal development as the antidote for our suffering health. In a clinical sense, drugs arise as the answer to everything that ails us. "We possess the illusion that we have just found an effortless shortcut to restoring our health, one with few or no adverse consequences, due to the the lack of relationship and detailed explanation of both the benefits and the fearful side effects of drugs" (Saputo & Belitsos, 2009).

Whether pursuing leadership, excellence, or more optimal health, adversity will always be present. Life will always pose challenges and circumstances that will disrupt our comfort zones.

The choices of attitude and of action in response to the discomfort determine the probability of success and influence.

You want to win? Respond to your adversity with integrity. Lock in, and be resolved. Seeking short term solutions, seeking what is easy, and seeking others who justify our passive decisions will deter character development.

What we seek when discomfort attacks our status quo is important.

Excellence has its roots here, in your response to adversity. What your habitual response is, and your effort moving forward despite the hardship can have a big impact towards success and towards health.

The choice is yours.

Embrace the suck.

CHAPTER 13

SUFFER WITH A SMILE

 Suffering. It is a bit of a dramatic word. Its potency elicits a harsh sense of discomfort. Forms of suffering in the world today have little resemblance to the suffering experienced in primitive times. However, it seems like a fitting term to describe the current plight of our health. "Most Americans gain a few pounds every year and rarely notice. Those few pounds lead to the growth rate of obesity. This translates directly into related ailments such as type 2 diabetes, heart disease, high blood pressure, and arthritis" (Olson, 2011, p. 191). We have been fading progressively from health, and our decline was been slow enough to go almost unnoticed. Both positive and negative lifestyle choices require habit, the bad habits we have adopted do not reveal their negative impact until time reveals the damage. Then we realize that we are suffering.

 Our own suffering has been a work in the making.

 Contributors to the onset of declining health and increasing diagnoses of preventable ailments include a fast paced society, advancements of technology, developments of pharmaceuticals, and convenience. Convenience - instant gratification - is a major culprit that plummets us toward bad habits. What is readily available for our consumption or use typically replaces personal effort. Speaking in terms of health attainment, we seek fast results and instant fixes. We want to be healthy, but we also want to exert as little effort as possible.

We desire to marry the most minimal of effort to the most massive of results.

Are we serious?

Health is a product of lifestyle. Lifestyle is not established in a day. Health, therefore, cannot be established in a day either. But we expect that with one or two choices that are outside our typical lifestyle, we can alter our current state of health - which has been a product of habitual lifestyle choices.

An extra serving of broccoli a week, one REALLY good workout, a 4 week program with a personal trainer, a 30 day diet trend... We place overreaching expectations on a temporary stimulus to "undo" lifestyle patterns built upon convenience.

We aren't actually willing to give up our lifestyle in order to change our course.

So when the temporary stimulus doesn't work (why we put so much faith in these, I'll never know), we give up. We say that whatever we chose as our "stimulus" is ineffective, not worth it, and a waste.

So we go back to our lifestyle of poor choices, feeling defeated. We tried to fix it, right? We gave "health" a chance, right?

For being an incredibly advanced society, we are incredibly naive.

Let's get real.

Your lifestyle determines your health.

Your habits determine your lifestyle.
Your choices determine your habits.
Your choices are your responsibility.
Own it.

The general pursuit of healing and optimal health with little sense of responsibility holds a deeper sense of failure than a lack of daily physical activity. Americans' physical health is failing.

On a more somber note, Americans are becoming progressively soft and mentally weak.

We lack the spine to stand up for our very own health.

And we are the ones to blame.

"We have become comfortable relying on an incomplete model of science and medicine to solve our health issues and have relinquished much of our personal responsibility to live a healthy lifestyle and build an ecologically sustainable world" (Saputo & Belitsos, 2009, p. 86).

By relinquishing our personal responsibility, we have no one to blame for physical suffering other than ourselves.

However, suffering can be a modality that contains limitless power. In previous chapters, mental toughness amidst adversity was shown to impact health. Returning to the foundational themes of excellence and success, let's look at how we can improve our health and halt suffering in its tracks.

Let's take ownership of our suffering health; let's take ownership to embrace a courageous attitude. Let's lock in to what is difficult. Let's deny cultural trends of instant gratification. Let's de-throne convenience in our lifestyle. Let's use our time and our energy to do what is most beneficial for our health status and attainment. Let's have the courage to change what we BELIEVE, and how we ACT to gain the most full assimilation of health into our lifestyle.

We begin through simple choices.

Begin a gratitude journal.

Smile more.

Exercise every day.

Eat good food.

Drink water.

"Defend your physical being with simple yet intentional choices regarding health diet, adequate sleep, limit toxic exposures, pursue a positive emotional and spiritual state" (Saputo & Belitsos, 2009, p. 171). As we do these things repeatedly, we begin to change our lifestyle. Thus, we move away from the status of suffering.

Confront the suffering of your body. Stand up against the instant gratification trends that hasten suffering. Start with a choice of action, and repeat it. A proven method (through personal experience) to improve physical well-being is to perform a pull-up, or at least hang from a bar. "One of the first things that pull-ups improves is our grip strength. This is important because it has a direct relationship with our longevity, as revealed through research studies that correlate strong grip to shorter hospital stays and better overall physical functioning" (Milner, 2019).

Trying to put forth minimal effort and maximize health?

Learn and practice pull-ups.

Best bang for your fitness buck!

There might be an ounce of effort, and maybe a bead of sweat involved. Yikes. Brace yourself. Practicing and habitually working on a pull-up might not be easy.

It appears as though a simple pull-up can decrease the suffering and failing of our personal health. The exercise itself is physical - chin over the bar on the way up, elbows extended on the way down. Simple. But pull-ups aren't exactly "popular" or "fun" in general (I am the anomaly). There might be a little discomfort with practicing pull-ups. But as we wrestle with the effort invested to train pull-ups on a consistent basis, let us also wrestle with the effort invested to become better leaders through our *personal* challenges. "You have two choices when confronting a challenge: shrink away from it or fight" (Zigarelli, 2011, p. 208). The link between physical health and our attitudes towards challenges is an aspect of character.

It's how leaders develop, grow, and gain influence.

We have discussed this previously. Physical and internal development affect every aspect of health. Which is reflected in our ability to be human and to exude influence. But this is proven through scientific literature. "Success in any one of these areas [various components of health] begins to affect all the others too. Improve your health and you improve your relationships; work on your personal development and you have an impact on your career. Everything affects everything else" (Olson, 2011, p. 110).

Buried deep within our general suffering as a society, each one of us has a subjective view suffering due to our personal experiences. It is important to note than my own establishment of suffering might be insignificant to another person. Putting aside the ego and refusing to judge each other's view of suffering is important if we truly value human association.

This is imperative. Perception of suffering is exclusively one's own. Yet, the suffering that we all encounter in various mechanisms is an incredible catalyst towards the development of purpose and of influence. We cannot overcome suffering without relationship. We cannot overcome without a purpose towards others. We cannot conquer without love.

"Suffering in and of itself is meaningless; we give our suffering meaning by the way in which we respond to it. Life is meaningful and we must learn to see life as meaningful despite our circumstances. In some way, suffering ceases to be suffering at the moment it finds a meaning, such as the meaning of a sacrifice. The captivity experience was seen [perceived] as a growth experience, 'I know that without the suffering, the growth that I have achieved would have been impossible'. Even if one cannot change the situation that causes the suffering, he can still choose his own attitude" (Frankl, 2006).

Frankl wrote these words as a prisoner in captivity, a victim of the Holocaust. He withstood and persevered experiences that we cannot venture to imagine. No description of "suffering" can illustrate the hardships he experienced. His ability to find and to evaluate meaning and purpose in life while in the midst of bitter suffering is one to be emulated. How did he find meaning amidst such suffering?
He viewed his suffering as an opportunity.
His meaning was that to support, encourage, and to love the victims around him, sharing in his suffering. He embraced a perception towards his suffering that allowed him an internal condition to believe in hope.
He was resolved to encourage the men around him towards life and freedom, regardless of how unlikely life and freedom appeared.

Love and hope were priorities, and held purpose.

The suffering we endure is a platform, and successful leaders view it as a moment to be seized. As soon as we choose to view suffering as an opportunity, as something other than negative or meaningless or burdensome, it suddenly can become meaningful.

Suffering can become a venue to overcome. To rise up, and to roar loudly, even if we are feeling meek and small on the inside.

A lion cub has a squeaky little roar, but once he matures, the roar becomes authoritative.

You must mature and practice your roar, before it may command an audience.

One must practice in a feeble state to move from it and towards a state of commanding authority.

Roar.

Believe that your suffering has meaning; it is an opportunity.

It can become a pathway to achieve, and to actualize a sense of accomplishment through a newfound perception.

Once an attitude is taken towards suffering, suffering produced by external circumstances beyond our control, growth and influence are granted. The way in which you choose responsibility to overcome the suffering for a greater purpose and meaning is the gauge of influence and the determinant of developing excellence. "There is one quality which one must possess to win, and that is definiteness of purpose, the knowledge of what one wants, and a burning desire to possess it" [Napoleon Hill] (Olson, 2011, p. 118).

Suffering should not have the power to downgrade your resolve of meaning or purpose.

Do not give it that power.

Every person has the choice to respond towards suffering. How we choose to bear our burdens also carries implications towards relationship and human interaction. Encouragement during times of uncertainty and strife can serve to increase the sense of purpose and of meaning. Throughout *"A Man's Search for Meaning"* the theme of suffering was a constant reality. Death was ever-present. However, Frankl's focus was not directed towards the suffering, but towards his focus to prioritize the way in which he found meaning .

"It is a question of attitude that one takes towards life's challenges and opportunities, both large and small. A positive attitude enables a person to endure suffering and disappointment as well as enhance enjoyment and satisfaction – negative attitude with undermine and diminish satisfaction. Those that remember that it is often through an exceptionally difficult external situation which gives man the opportunity to grow spiritually beyond himself" (Frankl, 2006, p. 60).

The choice to embrace a positive attitude is reflected through action. The power of an action rooted in attitude despite difficulty is unquantifiable. This power is evident, because it is a catalyst to provoke others to rise above their suffering as well. "The immediate influence of behavior is always more effective than that of words" (Frankl, 2006, p. 80).

The value of encouragement increases exponentially when difficulty and discomfort are present. When encouragement is the last thing we want to do - or *feel* like doing - is typically when it holds the most power.

The environment in which we act despite emotions showcases the resolve of our identity, attitude, behavior, and responsibly.

It presents an opportunity to actualize purpose for ourselves directed towards others in love.

"Attitude is a little thing that makes a big difference" [Winston Churchill] (Olson, 2011, p. 80).

In fact, I believe it makes all the difference.

CHAPTER 14

NEETURE

Nature. It's pretty neat. It's the neatest actually. Of all the unassuming and common elements of life, nature is by far the coolest. I am kinda a nature nerd. I love it. It's just beautiful and amazing. And of course the science of nature just adds to its magnificence. Photosynthesis, cloud formation, atmospheric changes, and frequencies of light and sound are just a few phenomena of nature. But there are some incredible scientific phenomena of nature that need no science in order to appreciate. Majestic mountains, powerful precipitation, colorful leaves, wildlife, frosty grass, warm sunshine, sounds of insects, cool refreshing air, berries and vegetables, volcanoes, serene lakes tucked between mountains, jagged coastlines, rainless deserts, colorful fall leaves…..nature is all around.

Creation offers nature freely.

Nature and the life it possesses take many forms. We miss many of them; or fail to appreciate them. We take many for granted. How often do we stop to literally and figuratively "smell the roses"? We appreciate the sound of the mighty ocean when we are on vacation. We appreciate mountains when we have orchestrated a camping trip to escape stress. We admire the crisp temperatures of fall and the colorful changes of trees in tandem with yummy pumpkin flavored drinks (and with the justification of warmth to wear baggy clothes). When we finally choose to acknowledge nature has no bearing over its ever-present availability to be recognized. Its impact can be appreciated every day. Yet few of us harness its power. It is freely offered; and it constantly invites. Its voice is drowned by the other voices we have chosen to value more.

Nature is amazing - the power reserved in it is unfathomable. Consider the power of the sun and the electrical charges of a lightening storm.

The power of nature can actually serve to save us. Why else do we find so much gratification from being near massive mountains, or the crashing waves of the ocean?

Nature is a concealed force behind who I am and my orientation towards life. I would even say that it is an aspect of my identity.

It's as though it is always there inspire me, to revive my spirit, to initiate gratitude - and it never asks for acknowledgement.

It never seeks anything from me. Yet I have gained life from it. The force of nature - completely independent of success, failure, politics, relationship, social norms - has fed my very soul. Nature is created with purpose, as am I. Yet it has no worries, fears, or cares. It has been created to exist within a system of energy that progresses without interference from humans. And as a human, my body too has been created to function as a biological system. But I can think, feel, and love - unlike plants and animals and rocks.

I am grateful for nature.

I am grateful that it operates independently of human advancement. Technology and medicine mean nothing to the commanding Redwoods of the Pacific Northwest.

I am in awe of the beauty and the function of the natural environment that surrounds me. It reminds me how truly small that I am. It reminds me that my cares, concerns, and my preoccupations really have little meaning. I am humbled by the gift of nature; it is given and operates freely for my benefit. And I have done absolutely nothing to deserve its gift of life. It indicates that there is a greater power, a greater essence that has provided its life. I owe nature, its design, its intricacies, and its unfathomable relationship to life to a Creator. The same One who orchestrated the organization of the Alps is the same One who initiated cellular function of our bodies with just a breath. I stand in awe of this One - the Author of all life.

Nature has brought me a sense of awareness to life. I'm not a radical free spirit (but please recycle, don't litter, and try to save trees when possible). I do love and desire to conserve and protect and take care of the outdoor environment. I believe it is a task given to all of us as humans from the Creator. I want my effort and my appreciation of nature to inspire others to seek its preservation too.

I love the outdoors. It's part of who I am, and I cannot do without it. I need trees. I need pine needles and leaves. I need grass and desert sand. I need open skies and dense canopies of brush. I need jagged massive boulders and serene transcendental lakes. I need light from the sun and from brilliant stars.

Just get me outdoors.

Throughout my childhood and into my high school career, my orientation towards life was organically (no pun intended) outdoors. I lived in the country, amidst small towns nestled among farmland, mountains, and woodland.

The way of life wasn't easy, and I was immersed in a blue collar environment. The environment around me created the career orientation of the residents of these small towns. Farmers, mechanics, construction workers, electricians and plumbers were numerous, and their jobs depended heavily upon seasonal changes. Each season offered its own characterization; beneficial to some occupations and a hindrance to others.

Each season brought the area around me specific natural phenomenons. Spring was characterized by wet, sloppy, muddy soil that served to be the pre-requisite for the most beautiful of flowers and a pronounced emergence of green buds. Warm and sloppy spring gave way to summer, which was hot and humid. Fall - probably the countryside's most awe inspiring seasons- manifested cool crisp mornings, the most radiant of foliage and smells of changing leaves, and the indulgence of apples, pumpkins, and cozy comforts as the temperatures steadily dropped. Winters in the countryside were indeed beautiful, as snowfalls would smoothly blanket the ground. As much as cold temperatures were sometimes less than pleasant, warm clothing and warm company were fitting respite.

Each season also had corresponding outdoor activities. Springtime was a period to clean up the landscape around the house with whatever winter had ravaged. Springtime was the opportunity for me and my family to plant, clean, and organize the acres of land around my home. The backside of my house was heavily wooded. The woods was beautiful, but I remember spending hours of shaping up and tidying what nature had dumped in the gutters and on the lawn. In the heat of summer, I remember weeding the garden, push mowing my huge yard, cherry picking and green bean snipping, and landscaping. These chores were interwoven with sports, events, and weekend adventures. Recreational soccer games and practices took up weeknights and weekend afternoons. Camping trips and cabin trips filled weekends not consumed by sports. Weekdays were spent chipping away at the to-do list and preparing for the next adventure of summer.

Horseback riding lessons were also included on the list of activities. Summer riding was much more fun than riding in the winter, and I am convinced that the horses enjoyed summer trail rides too.

Other than vacuuming, dusting, and cleaning toilets, little of the to-do list occurred indoors. Chores and activities were done outdoors.

As summer trickled into the fall, soccer season became my main priority. Farming and hunting were central priorities for the locals; as both the harvest and the visions of bagging the biggest deer trophies dominated the topics of conversation. Along with the fun outdoor activities of the fall season, the seasonal chores of country life required attention. Chopping down dead trees for firewood was high on the priority list- winters were cold and the wood stove needed fuel. I spent many days with my family loading and stacking firewood. Several iterations into the mountain to chop, throw, dump, carry, and stack firewood were necessary to keep the house warm during the upcoming chilly months. We loaded the pickup truck to its maximum capacity with firewood, then drove it down the mountain. After dumping all the pieces in the yard, we took the time to stack each and every piece of firewood.

Hundreds of pieces.

Carry the piece, stack the piece, walk back to the pile.

Repeat.

Until the dumped pile of pieces was re-established in neat stacks, we worked.

It was "forced family fun"... but in retrospect, wood-stacking actually served as wonderful family bonding.

And I can still toss firewood quite efficiently, and I enjoy it.

Firewood stacking and raking the yard consumed lots of time after school. The yard was huge, and once it was covered with leaves, it became a chore to rake. Several days were dedicated to leaf blowing and raking. The process was long and tedious. However, there was the promise of fun. Raking a huge pile of leaves resulted in hours upon hours of leaf jumping, and calloused hands were definitely worth it! The large pile of leaves raked from the yard was traditionally gathered under our home-made rope swing. The rope swing offered the perfect method of transport from solid ground into the welcoming mound of soft leaves. Over and over my siblings and I would cling to the rope, swing over the leaves, release our grip, and be swallowed by the huge mound of leaves. After hours of raking, jumping and laughing finished the day. But the removal of leaves from my hair was an additional chore that was always more painful than expected.

The fall season offered both beauty and flavor. My siblings and I would go to a local orchard and select bushels of apples. The most delicious of apples. The numerous ripe and juicy golden delicious apple were to be made into fresh applesauce. Making applesauce took an entire day - it transformed the kitchen into systematic chaos. The apples were washed, heated on the stovetop until soft, placed into the hand churner, and the sauce was produced and collected! The sweet sticky warm applesauce was ladled into glass mason jars. It was sealed and canned, so that it could be enjoyed at any time. To this day, fresh applesauce, freshly picked golden delicious apples, and apple picking bring joy to my soul. My affection for crunchy, sweet, tart, and juicy apples is shared with soft, subtle, uniquely nutty pumpkins. Fall seasons create opportunity for these flavors to take many forms - warm beverages, savory main dishes and soups, attention grabbing side dishes, and sweet desserts.

There are few apple or pumpkin flavored things that I am not a fan of.

I'm one of those people who enjoys pumpkin things year round.

I love pumpkins.

And apples.

All the time.

The arrival of winter brought cold, snowfall, and ice. There was much time dedicated to shoveling snow, clearing footpaths, and defrosting windshields. Snow brought challenges to daily function, but it also brought adventure and fun (of course). Snowfall and cold temperatures were essential factors for sledding down my slick driveway and down the hundreds of yards of the sloping farmland. My house was the venue for countless sledding parties. Parked trucks and SUVs bordered the driveway while saucers and runner sleds (the old ones with the metal tracks, wicked fast!) and toboggans and even large slabs of plastic served to give us the greatest thrills! We would speed down the slippery snow and ice, hardly in control of our sleds. Between the driveway and the farmland, many memories were created on sleds; freezing temperatures at night didn't deter us. In fact, sled parties were only possible at night, when the cooler night temperatures caused the snow to be a bit more slick. With only the moon to light our "path", blind sledding adventures brought out our inner adrenaline junkies. Fatigue and cold toes were the only reasons we ever went indoors; but the enticing promise of hot chocolate and snacks made going indoors seem justified. Piles of snowpants, jackets, gloves, and hats filled the entryway of the house. Pairs of boots were lined up in front of the wood stove to dry. Those sledding parties and winter nights were the most fun. And resulted in the many memories, and a trip or two to the emergency room. But everyone survived, and now have great stories to share!

In the winter months, the living room area in front of the wood stove looked more like a Salvation Army or Goodwill - random winter clothing scattered about in no organized fashion, with gloves and socks and pants and thermal layers laid out all over the floor and strewn up on clothing racks.

As I look back at my years before college, I realize that my life was spent outside, doing things.

My memories really don't include indoor activities.

My family and I were always outdoors.

I was constantly on the move, in nature.

It was a way of life.

Being outdoors was normal, and the orientation towards the outdoors was ordinary. Not only was is commonplace, but it required no effort to manifest.

There was just no reason to be indoors.

Technology was not as present or as integral to everyday life as it is today; and thus, there was no distraction to doing things outdoors. There was too much to be done. Everyday life required "to-do's" to be accomplished outside.

Jobs and careers were done outside. Community and relationship were formed performing tasks and jobs. Which by necessity and by nature (puns), occurred outdoors.

The theme of camaraderie with performing outdoor activities is what made my small town childhood experiences so meaningful, and so full. What had to be accomplished outdoors was done relationally. My siblings and I were rarely apart; my family members and friends took credit for things that were accomplished because we worked together. There was rarely a solo effort on any endeavor or task. There was satisfaction in a work completed as a team.

It was a beautifully simple form of productivity, and simple form of building relationship.

With the help of others, things got done.

And relationships were formed through hard work. Effort invested in the task revealed the care we had towards each other. I worked hard to get a job done, knowing that my investment mattered. If I didn't work hard on a shared task with my siblings, they could justify also investing partial effort. It was a mutual understanding- if I work hard, then the effort I invest will overflow towards my siblings' work ethic too. And thus, relationship was build and jobs got done.

The mentality was simple.

Go outside, do what needs doing without complaint, and then have fun when the task is complete. Even before afternoon soccer events, I was required to do my chores. Push mowing, weeding, raking, stacking firewood... certain tasks were pre-requisites for soccer games. The chores didn't cause me to be tired before soccer. All I knew was that I wanted to play soccer. The task, no matter how "tough", wasn't too difficult or too tiring. I wouldn't allow it. I wanted to play the game I loved. I loved the sport, I loved the competition.

In order to play, I had to get the list of chores done. And done well. There was no question about it, there was never any caveat to completion. So, I did the tasks required of me. And then I was allowed to exhaust myself on the soccer field. What a perfect day.

I look back fondly at this structure; for it taught me the value of getting hard work done in its fullest completion before one is to enjoy the fruits of labor.

I have already explained the value of doing things, and the value of mindset behind physical effort. Physical effort and the power of the mind are components of health, as discussed previously. However, there is an environmental effect upon health, through physical effort and the power of the mind that needs to be explored.

Seasonal changes and nature itself, physical exercise, and the human mind are integrated.

At this point, this should cause no surprise.

My orientation towards exercise and towards nature plays a direct role on my health and wellbeing.

I am an athlete, and I seek optimal performance and physiological adaptations. My performance is graded by any accomplishment that I am able to achieve. Regardless of my athletic aspirations, I believe that exercise, or activity, performed outdoors increases health parameters. Simply being around a rural environment, where many jobs are dependent upon physical effort and exercise, causes the pursuit of health to be engrained into lifestyle.

Does activity being performed outdoors offer increased benefits to health and wellbeing in addition to the established benefits of exercise? What role does being outdoors, in naturally occurring life, have on us, especially if we exercise outdoors?

I turned to the research, and indeed, nature does have an influence on our health.

Crazy.

A study performed in the UK evaluated several modalities of activity performed outside to analyze the relationship of health and "green exercise". The results of the study revealed that exercise outside can result in mental health benefits. They found that "self esteem and mood were found to affected by "green exercise"; regardless of type, intensity, or duration of exercise" (Pretty, et al., Green Exercise in the UK Countryside: Effects on Health and Psychological Well-Being, and Implications for Policy and Planning, 2007).

The authors affirmed that a natural environment can promote good health from a variety of disciplines. Furthermore, people with low self esteem can benefit from exercise, but even more so with exercise performed outside. (Pretty, et al., Green Exercise in the UK Countryside: Effects on Health and Psychological Well-Being, and Implications for Policy and Planning, 2007).

"Activities performed at neighborhoods and rural areas vary based upon physical, social, and cultural factors. However, the behavioral and lifestyle changes that can occur as a result of habitual practice have implications over emotional and mental wellbeing of the population. Green exercise could reduce the common state of human suffering that includes obesity, anxiety, and depression" (Pretty, et al., Green exercise in the UK countryside: Effects on health and psychological well-being, and implications for policy and planning, 2007).

"It can be used as a vehicle to drive behavioral change and ensure a more inclusive approach to health, and used as an intervention offered to those suffering from mental disorders and resulting behavioral conduct" (Barton, Bragg, Wood, & Pretty, 2016).

As mentioned in previous chapters, the root cause of many mental health diagnoses, such as depression and anxiety, can be found outside the brain and successfully treated (Nikogosian, 2019).

"Higher rates of physical activity and lower incidence of obesity have been associated with regular physical activity, time spent outdoors, and access to green space. Individuals with easy physical and cultural access to natural settings are three times as likely to engage in physical activity, experience less mental distress and have overall better wellbeing"(Barton, Bragg, Wood, & Pretty, 2016). "Nature contact is not only a multisensory experience, exposing individuals to sunlight to aid vitamin D production, but it also provides a space to be active, mindful, socially interactive, develop a sense of place and attachments to both people and places" (Barton, Bragg, Wood, & Pretty, 2016).

How much more evidence do we need to motivate us to simply go outside?

Anxiety, depression, obesity, and other chronic diseases can have one common treatment.

Exercise outside.

Simple. And free.

Why are we allowing ourselves to degenerate, to suffer, to prefer lifestyles that drive us far from a state of health?

We fail to take ownership.

We fail to be responsible for ourselves.

We fail to own our choices.

We fail to value and prioritize health and influence only gained through hard work.

We fail to be resolved.

We fail to identify ourselves based upon a solid foundation.

We rob ourselves of joy by comparing ourselves.

We fail to value relationship over quantifiable measures, and thus fail to embrace full meaning of life.

We fail to love.

I'll continue with science, in case you still aren't convinced.

Research has validated that activity outdoors is beneficial for mental and biological function. Regular outdoor activity can help to mitigate some various suboptimal lifestyle choices, such as diet. "We all know that Americans are increasingly overfed, and yet undernourished, and that obesity, diabetes, heart disease, cancer, and mental health problems are linked to diet"(Saputo & Belitsos, 2009, p.225). Can going outside prevent metabolic syndrome? Not directly. But it can increase other factors of health to minimize the detriment of a poor diet.

We are surrounded by nature that offers health, yet we exist in individual pockets of ignorance as we try to obtain health from other sources.

As we stand or sit at our desks.

As we do our WOD at the gym.

As we socialize around a sports bar.

Our patterns of life, no matter how well intended, occur indoors.

Cultures that exist in rural environments have reported correlations between a disease free state and quality of life, specifically, happiness (Yang, 2017).

Ironic? I think not.

We cannot be so naive to believe that the lack of disease confirms a condition of health. "Achieving good mental health is not just a reflection of the absence of disease or disability. It comprises a balance between self-satisfaction, independence, capability and competency, achieving potential, and coping well with stress and adversity" (Barton & Pretty, What is the best dose of nature and green exercise for improving mental health? A multi-study analysis., 2010).

"Optimizing our health is unique to each person and goes beyond only ensuring the absence of disease" (Nikogosian, 2019).

Peeling back the "optimization of health" to its very core, developing our internal selves, which directly influences the function of our minds and our bodies, stems from the fulfillment of our individual purpose.

Read that sentence again.

Write it down in the gratitude journal that you are going to start.

Each of us has a unique purpose, a unique calling, and a special meaning that only we can manifest. "We are not a product of heredity and environment, not a result of biological, psychological, and sociological conditions. We are not a pawn and victim of outer influences or inner circumstances. Everyone has his own specific vocation or mission in life to carry out a concrete assignment which demands fulfillment. The primary motivation in life is our search for meaning: the "will to meaning" – as opposed to the will to pleasure or the will to power. Meaning must be fulfilled by each of us individually; only then does it achieve a significance which will satisfy our unique will to meaning" (Frankl, 2006).

I have no more angles to approach this topic.

Your identity and your unique meaning matter.

Practice ownership of your identity.

Since practice and repetition and habit are crucial to health, excellence, and leadership, I'll proceed to reiterate the importance of our soul development.

Our internal selves, our self image, and our interactions with nature are linked to our ability to function as biological beings. "Human beings are an inseparable combination of body, mind, emotion, and spirit, as these are embedded in society, culture, and the universe" (Saputo & Belitsos, 2009, p. 23). Internal self matters, in relationship to each other and our expression of meaning towards others. But how much do we really care about other people compared to how much we care about ourselves? The answer to that question can be answered on an individual level. But the sad truth about health is that we have manipulated "health" to have a financial implication, instead of life and function implication. We have made it a system, instead of a holistic connection of choices to the ability to live life.

If self esteem and mood are improved due to activity in the outdoors, why is "green exercise" not valued? Why aren't we doing it? Why is it not prescribed more by medical professionals? Telling patients to go outside, and to exercise outside, doesn't make the doc any money....

Why do we give in to excuses and sustain poor health?

Are the keys to success just too simple for us to actually take confidence in?

Does it disrupt our comfort zone?

Do we value what other people think SO much that we are willing to permit a lack of health?

Regardless the reason (or excuse) that we deny exercise outdoor and deny positive and simple lifestyle choices to aid in our pursuit of health, we are only ones to blame.

We have complete ownership to step outside.

We all have the access and the capability to expose ourselves to a natural environment.

Exercise mode, intensity, and duration are of less importance than the simple exposure of nature. The impact it has on mood, self esteem, and biological function is undeniable.

It's simple. Nature is all around us.

Take a moment to soak it in, as it is always there to benefit you.

Make the choice. Exposures through repeated and consistent action, seemingly so simple, can increase your ability to embrace health and defend your immune system.

Seems like a familiar theme that tracks all the way back to Chapter 1.

Health and excellence are linked.

Health and nature are linked.

Therefore, nature and excellence are linked.

To step towards excellence, one must value that which they cannot control.

Value the lack of control.

Nature is uncontrollable, as are circumstances; thus, to embrace nature and embrace circumstance welcomes capability to affect our bodies and our souls.

Experiencing nature and experiencing circumstances cause us to respond. The experiences themselves are outside our control.

But our responses are totally in our control.

Choose to value life around you.

Choose patterns that are saturated in integrity and authenticity.

Serve people. Be grateful. Exercise. Love others.

Act in a purpose that transcends quantification; your purpose towards fellow humans and your purpose towards excellence matters.

Act in a purpose grounded in love and gratitude.

This generates life.

A cycle of life begins in your heart.

Act to inspire life in others.

Nature and its benefit to our very souls is waiting to be seized; shift your attention towards it.

Rake some leaves.

Cannonball into a lake.

Sled down a hill.

Weed a flowerbed.

Be a natural and excellent human.

Love.

CHAPTER 15

DILLY DILLY

You've made it this far! Thank you for putting forth the effort of leafing through these pages. Thank you for reading words from my heart and from my individual perspective. Thank you for allowing your imagination to join me as I recounted some past experiences. Thank you for continuing to make it this far, despite my over energetic feelings about corn, dirt, fitness, and rustic cabins.

I honor the time and mental effort that you have put forth browsing these pages. I will keep this final chapter short and sweet, and to the point.

I'm short, so I guess it fits.

Sweet.... Well sometimes I attempt to be.

To the point, that is me to a T.

This final chapter wraps up all of the themes I have brought forth into one. This theme is what I have deemed **pondition**. Pondition is a word that combines *position* and *condition*. Pondition is a theme that lies beneath all the elements of influence, success, excellence, and leadership.

Before I explain how pondition works, I will reveal pondition in my current life.

My stories have all been in the past, some more recent than others. I will now share my current situation, and how my pondition is expressed.

I am recovering from my foot surgery. I must wear a boot full time, and I am allowed to walk on it and adequately cause the bone to become "stressed" in order to adapt and become stronger. I am able to work on a limited basis, as I am only confident driving a few miles. I am able to use my energy, my education, and my love for people a few hours a week with personal training. I am trying to increase cardiovascular and strength based fitness, as my functional capabilities slowly return. I am struggling through my nutrition, as I am mentally working to fuel my body properly and to encourage healing. My attitudes and mindset around nutrition are shifting slowly, it is a much harder process than I had ever imagined. I am struggling with disordered eating. My actions towards food reflect an improper relationship between my thoughts and nutrition. Being a high achieving elite athlete, and one who understands science of nutrition, I am challenged with nutrition habits in light of both *what I know* combined with *who I am*. This challenge has been confounded incredibly with my injury and recovery. The injury has caused training to take a drastic shift, and therefore my attitude towards nutrition shifted too. And I am still working though the relationship I have with nutrition.

I am an alumni mentor of a current MWS player. This is an incredible honor and privilege for me, as I am able to pour encouragement into her, and at the same time, remain connected to the MWS program than has impacted me so deeply.

I am eager to soon begin my NSCA Assistantship with the 10thSFG at Fort Carson in the new year, mere weeks away. Before that time comes when I must relocate towards the Army base, I reside near the Denver area. I have treasured the relationships that I have made in my time here. The adults around me have surrounded me with love, encouragement, support, and meaning. They have allowed me into their lives and have revealed to me their wisdom and learning. Since I am new to Colorado, and will be in several temporary situations for the upcoming phase of life, I don't really have an established friend group. This reality is actually a blessing, for it allows me to appreciate in a more comprehensive way the relationships of friends and family back east in PA. Although nearly 1600 miles away, they are close to my heart.

These relationships are strong, through conscious and delegated effort.

I will spend Thanksgiving and Christmas here in Colorado, with some of my neighbors and new friendships. I am looking forward to a holiday season of new experiences in a new environment.

That is my current life situation.

Pondition is a combination of position and condition.
I'll break down my pondition.

My *position* in life is this: I am not in a full time job, but soon to begin an incredible experience at Fort Carson.

I am so blessed to serve some wonderful people as their personal trainer. I am healing from injury and somewhat limited in function. I am new to Colorado, and am establishing relationships and connections. I am struggling to pay off grad school loans and medical bills, confounded by being unable to work over the past few months.

My *condition* in life is this: I am thankful for the family and friends who have offered so much support - physical, emotional, financial, social, and spiritual. I am joyful to be able to be more functional than I was several weeks ago. I am blessed to see people around me, to appreciate humans and life. This appreciation and reliance on gratitude has filled my soul. Sometimes my heart yearns for my family back home, especially with my younger sister's recent engagement. Sometimes my spirit is dampened because I am unable to see my best friend, who just announced her pregnancy (woo!!!).

My position in life is based upon circumstances. My position in life is in flux, and can change at any given point in time. There is little about my position that I am in direct and universal control of. My *position* in life can threaten to hinder or alter my *condition* in life. But only if I allow it to have that power. My condition in life is the state of mind that I choose despite my current position in life. My condition operates independently from my position. My condition operates dependent upon my identity and immovable foundation of purpose.

My position may not always be up to me, but my condition is always up to me.

The level to which I allow position in life to alter my condition in life is pondition. My pondition, much like the continuum of health, is one that I take complete ownership of. I have worked hard to get here. The previous months of healing have been rough; they have been incredibly difficult from a variety of perspectives. However, my condition of joy and gratitude have risen to the surface, due to the strength of the Lord. His strength has enabled me to squash the threat of hopelessness and the attitude of impairment. Only by His strength, the condition of my soul is free and complete. I am no victim of circumstances. My soul is expectant of an unknown future as my heart rests in trust that the Lord has plans for me to prosper.

In general, we believe that our position directly influences our condition. The truth is, that mindset is an excuse. And it reflects lack of courage, and presence of weakness and fear. No position can force you to choose your personal condition. Evaluate what your position is in life. What are the external circumstances that shape how you approach your day to day? Now, evaluate your condition, taking into account your perception of those circumstances. What mindset do you approach the day with? How and why is your perspective manifested? Where do you base your condition, and how often do you allow that base to shift?

The answers to these questions will reveal your pondition.

An optimal pondition is one in which you have taken complete ownership of who you are, and your behavior that flows from meaning, regardless of your current position. An optimal pondition is one that compares position to no one, and to nothing; and is one that values and prioritizes love and relationship over all. An optimal pondition is one that has a focus driven not by performance or expectation, but by thankfulness, trust, and love.

The theme of pondition is a powerful undercurrent; it can be swift and lead an impactful, fulfilled, and satisfied life.

The secret to a condition being completely independent of position?

Your condition needs a solid foundation.

A condition with a foundation that can never and will never be shaken.

This foundation, the one that I have found to be infallible, immovable, and steadfast, is the Lord Jesus Christ.

Throughout my highest of highs, lowest of lows, kicking soccer balls in the dark and ugly crying, running my best races and achieving some crazy athletic feats, moving around the country, sifting through painful relationships and personal failures...my foundation has been built in trust and faith upon God. The various positions of life could only shake me if I allowed them to replace the only immovable foundation - Jesus.

He is the definition of love, and He has created me to reflect that love. I am here to overflow with love and joy. My source of these is Him; and He never fails. Therefore, if I truly am defined and found in Him, and trust wholeheartedly that His love for me is unconditional and unfathomable, then I am free to act in a way that reveals this same love that I am freely given. I am free to receive and to give grace to others. Nothing about what I personally accomplish here has significance; no, it is the way in which I show others my trust and faith in an all-powerful and all-knowing God. The way that I live as a reflection of the Lord results in life lived to the fullest. Hence, I am free. I can live in abandon to the cares of this world. I live as an example of love, with the purpose to serve others and claim nothing as my own.

I am not here for me. I am here to love. I am cared for by a God who loves me like crazy. He has never let me down. And He has promised to never let me down. He is my hope, my rock.

From this Rock, I can roar as loudly as I can. My roar is one that He delights in hearing. I roar with a sound that resounds towards souls. My roar is not dampened by my mistakes or my failures. Since my failures do not define me, they have no power over me. My roar is powerful because it is sourced by the King.

A lion with a booming roar is what you have within you. Only after you discover the source of the roar may you produce your own powerful roar. Once you discover it, it will shake the depths your soul; it will set you free. You will be free to love, to lead, to influence to a level beyond your dreams.

Roar.

EPILOGUE

A lion. Majestic and powerful. Fierce. Reserved until provoked. Leader of the pride. Effortlessly confident.

A lion can be a visual representation of my words. The stories told are all true, all recollections of adventures. My brief period here on earth has been rich of experiences and of learning. My journey thus far in life has already allowed me incredible opportunities to be influenced and to learn how to influence. Principles that bring about influence are ones that I am trying to integrate into my life. Excellence is a habit. My pursuit of excellence is always under my control. The power of my choices have allowed me to identify myself.

I am a lion.

I possess power without needing to say a word, or to purposefully demonstrate it.

I do not need to assert myself, my identity flows from my being.

I am meaningful.

I am a leader.

I am confident.

I am loved.

I hope that by sifting through my words and stories you can realize that you too are a lion. You can lead. You can be confident. You can be unconcerned with circumstances or perceptions around you. You can fulfill your meaning.

You ARE loved.

You have been assigned a great purpose, whether you realize it or not. You can be defined by a Love that is the source of life. It will never wane, never fade, never let you down. In fact, you have the potential to be so incredibly full of life that it spills over into the lives of everyone around you.

A lion doesn't need to roar for the pride to know who is in charge. A lion does not need to prove that he is strong and fierce. His countenance alone conveys his power.

You have nothing to prove, other than who you are, for yourself.

I am loved and defined by the One who created the lion. I am fulfilled, satisfied, and overflowing with a confidence of life the cannot be squelched. I hope in a future unknown to me, trusting fully in the One who loves me so much to guarantee my future. I rest in uncertainty, knowing that my power is finite and limited. My lack of certainly allows me to lean into the One whose power is limitless, and who knows my future. I can tap into that power if I release my grip on control, and fully trust Him. Knowing that I possess a power that is unquantifiable gives me confidence and hope. I embrace joy as a choice, eager to maximize it for the world to feel.

Join me.

I am not an island, and neither are you.

We are here for each other; to love the way in which we are loved.

Realizing the love that is unconditional, never failing, and never waning is my confidence. It is the platform from which I love others. The love I am identified by is the love the causes me to sacrifice and to serve others in the effort to show them how much they matter. You matter. You deserve love. You are loved.

Your inner lion is yearning to roar. Unleash it. Fill your lungs, fill your heart, with love. Trust. Abandon the need to control your own path ahead. Trust in the One that actually knows it all. Allow trust in Him and freedom to rush over your fears; let it fuel your purpose of love. Let it flood and overflow your soul. Roar so loudly because your heart is brimming over with love. Set your foundation on a source that never fails. Set your priorities on that which has a meaning beyond this world. And remain immovable to the cause of Love.

I stand humbly on a Rock.

"Therefore, my friends, do not be shaken. Remain steadfast and immovable. For you can be sure that the effort you exert for the Lord will not be in vain" ~ 1 Corinthians 15:58 (Holy Bible, 2011). Paraphrased from the NIV, this verse in the Bible is my favorite This verse is my mantra: I have the reference tattooed on my ribcage. It reminds me that as long as my efforts and prioritization in life are for the King, that I can progress in life confidently and with hope. Just in case I allow fears or anxiety an undue position in my heart, I have this reminder stamped in ink. It is always there to remind me and guide me back to the light and love that conquers all fears and redirects my focus.

Steadfast and immovable.

Defined by love.

Bibliography

1. (2019). (Dictionary.com Unabridged) Retrieved October 2019, from Dictionary.com: https://www.dictionary.com/browse/health
2. (2019). (Dictionary.com Unabridged) Retrieved October 2019, from Dictionary.com: https://www.dictionary.com/browse/resilience?s=t
3. Barton, J., & Pretty, J. (2010). What is the best dose of nature and green exercise for improving mental health? A multi-study analysis. Environmental Science and Technology, 44(10).
4. Barton, J., Bragg, R., Wood, C., & Pretty, J. (2016). Preface. In Green Exercise: Linking Nature, Health and Well-Being. London; New York: Routledge.
5. Bigliassi, M., León-Domínguez, U., Buzzachera, C., Barreto-Silva, V., & Altimari, L. (2015, February). How Does Music Aid 5km of Running? Journal of Strength and Conditioning Research, 29(2).
6. Cloud, D. H. (2014). Never Go Back: 10 Things You'll Never Do Again. Howard Books.
7. Frankl, V. E. (2006). Man's Search for Meaning. Beacon Press.
8. Goncalves, M. (2019, October 3). Keeping Faith During My Cancer Journey. Retrieved from The Epoch Times: https://www.theepochtimes.com/keeping-faith-during-my-cancer-journey_3096767.html
9. Holy Bible, New International Version®, NIV® Copyright ©1973, 1978, 1984, 2011 by Biblica, Inc.® Used by permission. All rights reserved worldwide.

10. Jenne, S. C.-C. (2019, October). Implementing Strength Training to Improve Ruck Marching Capacity. NSCA TSAC Report(55).

11. Ketler, A. (2016, April 8). Doctors Explan How Hiking ACtually Changes Our Brains. Retrieved November 2019, from Collective Evolution: https://www.collective-evolution.com/2016/04/08/doctors-explain-how-hiking-actually-changes-our-brains/?fbclid=IwAR1lT7rYgCpojXiVbI5V5r9ePOpxH15LYq266rxbiu-If9b7k6-pgEYWsFE

12. Milner, C. (2019, October 3). Why You Should Start Doing Pull-Ups . Retrieved from The Epoch Times: https://www.theepochtimes.com/why-you-should-start-doing-pull-ups_3096676.html

13. Nikogosian, A. (2019, October 3). A Wider Path to Wellness. Retrieved from The Epoch Times: https://www.theepochtimes.com/why-dont-i-feel-good_3094254.html

14. Olson, J. (2011). The Slight Edge: Turning Simple Disciplines Into Massive Success. Success Books.

15. Pretty, J., Peacock, J., Hine, R., Sellens, M., South, N., & Griffin, M. (2007). Green exercise in the UK countryside: Effects on health and psychological well-being, and implications for policy and planning. Journal of Environmental Planning and Management, 50(2), 211-231.

16. Pretty, J., Peacock, J., Hine, R., Sellens, M., South, N., & Griffin, M. (2007, March). Green Exercise in the UK Countryside: Effects on Health and Psychological Well-Being, and Implications for Policy and Planning. Journal of Environmental Planning and Management, 50(2), 211-231.

17. Saputo, L., & Belitsos, B. (2009). A Return to Healing: Radical Health Care Reform and the Future of Medicine. Origin Press.

18. Willink, J., & Babin, L. (2015). Extreme Ownership: How U.S Navy SEALs Lead and Win. 320: St. Martin's Press.

19. Yang, Y., Bekemeier, B., & Jongsan, C. (2017, March). Health-related Quality of Life and Related Factors among Rural Residents in Cambodia. Iranian Journal of Public Health, 46(3), 422-424.

20. Zigarelli, M. A. (2011). The Messiah Method. Xulon Press.

ABOUT THE AUTHOR

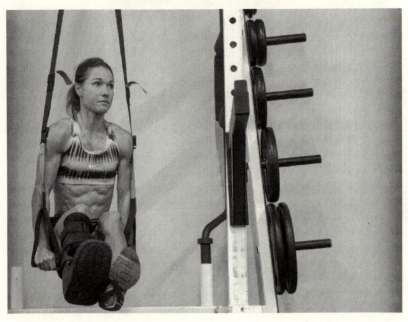

Regina Stump is an NCAA DIII Women's Soccer two-time National Champion (2011-2012) and current Elite Spartan Athlete and trail ultramarathoner. She aspires to one day complete a full Ironman. Her experiences as a collegiate athlete at Messiah College (PA) equipped her with a philosophical framework - to seize the opportunities of leadership and pursuit of excellence learned and broadly apply them. Competitive and driven, Regina desires her own work ethic, athletic pursuits, and conduct to reflect the power of influence, discipline, responsibility, and choice. The

power of love and purpose towards relationships source her energy and her motivations. She defines herself solely by love authored by Jesus Christ. Through love, Regina seeks to instill health and ownership to others. She believes that "the stronger society can grip onto personal responsibility, the stronger we are as biological and as relational beings. To serve others, to be grateful in all things, to value each other over ourselves is the template for fulfillment. Therefore, health is initiated within the heart and soul. It overflows into actions. And it finishes with a pull-up."

POWER LIES IN HEALTH.

HEALTH IS A FORCE.

YOU HAVE POWER.

FIERCE AND COURAGEOUS; WITH THE ROAR OF A LION.

Health evades our society. We seek and strive for health, for influence, for comfort, for identity, and success. We exhaust ourselves in this pursuit. We chase down the most attractive of methods to increase our health and to increase our positions in life. We chase it tirelessly; but dwindle with the onset of fear and futility.

The pages inside offer freedom; and hope. Open the cover and be revived. You need no validation for who you are, and your capability to lead with excellence, to be healthy, and to live each day with overwhelming purpose. The ordinary, the common, the seemingly trivial moments of life are moments where your power is forged.

Habits. Choices. Relationships. Here in lies the capability for your condition to supersede your position. Position varies. Condition is yours to seize. Seize the condition of your inner lion. Courageous and fierce, inspiring respect. Your power; your worth; your very being is meaningful. Believe it and act from it. Roar with confidence.

Read on; and become equipped for health, for leadership, and for success.

Made in the USA
Middletown, DE
14 October 2021